From Garden to Table

1500 Days of Fresh and Vibrant Vegan Delights with a 28-Day Meal Plan to Expand Your Culinary Horizon / Full Color Edition

Christina J. Williamson

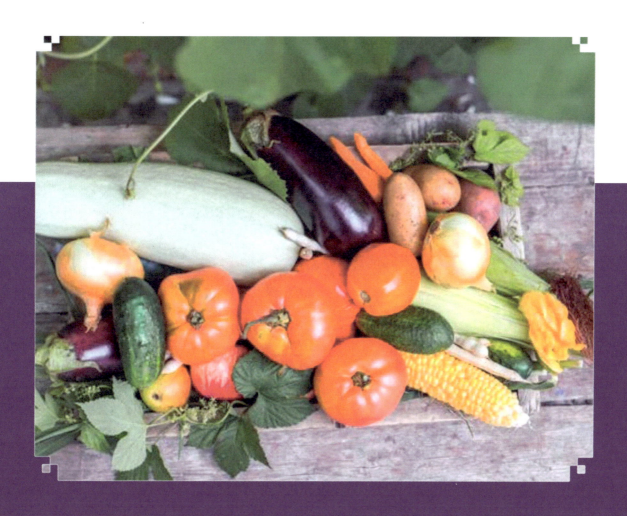

Copyright© 2024 By Christina J. Williamson Rights Reserved

This book is copyright protected. It is only for personal use. You cannot amend, distribute, sell, use, quote or paraphrase any part of the content within this book, without the consent of the author or publisher.

Under no circumstances will any blame or legal responsibility be held against the publisher, or author, for any damages, reparation, or monetary loss due to the information contained within this book, either directly or indirectly.

Disclaimer Notice:

Please note the information contained within this document is for educational and entertainment purposes only. All effort has been executed to present accurate, up to date, reliable, complete information. No warranties of any kind are declared or implied. Readers acknowledge that the author is not engaged in the rendering of legal, financial, medical or professional advice. The content within this book has been derived from various sources. Please consult a licensed professional before attempting any techniques outlined in this book.

By reading this document, the reader agrees that under no circumstances is the author responsible for any losses, direct or indirect, that are incurred as a result of the use of the information contained within this document, including, but not limited to, errors, omissions, or inaccuracies.

Editor: AALIYAH LYONS

Interior Design: BROOKE WHITE

Cover Art: DANIELLE REES

Food stylist: SIENNA ADAMS

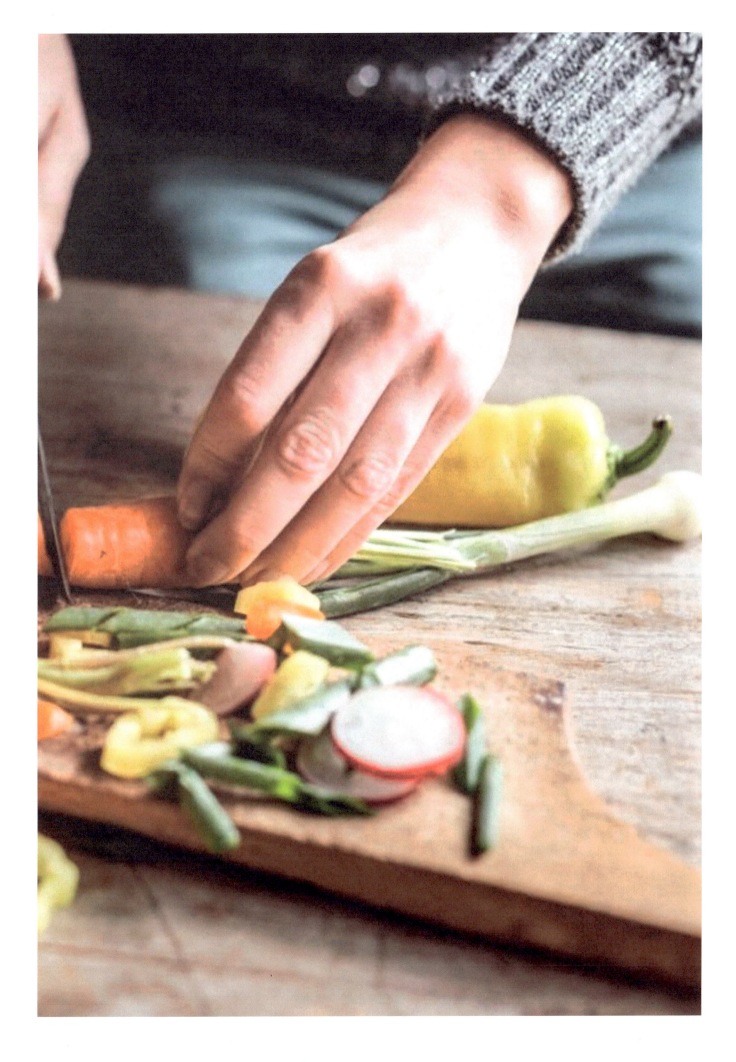

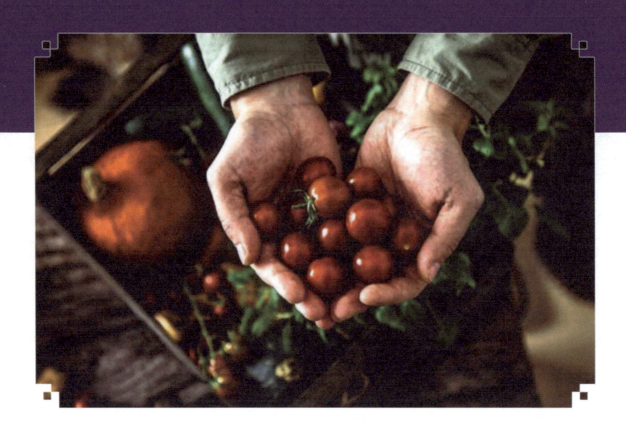

Table Of Contents

Introduction	1
Chapter 1	
Celebrating Your Vegan Journey	2
Principles and Benefits of Veganism	3
Stocking Your Vegan Kitchen	4
Q&As for Beginners	5
Chapter 2	
4-Week Meal Plan	7
Week 1	8
Week 2	9
Week 3	10
Week 4	11

Chapter 3	
Versatile Sauces and Fillings	13
Mexican Rice Filling	14
Cheesy Vegetable Sauce	15
Caesar-Style Dressing	15
Green Enchilada Sauce	16
Homemade Ketchup	16
Mango Salad Dressing	17
Garlic-Mushroom Sauce	17
Creamy Leek Sauce	18
Mild Harissa Sauce	18
Yellow Pepper Sauce	19
Buffalo-Style Barbecue Sauce	19
Chapter 4	

Breakfast and Brunch Creations 20
Strawberry Oatmeal 21
Easy Nonfat Garlic Bread 22
Cinnamon Donut Bites 23
Spring Breakfast Salad 23
Strawberry-Kiwi Chia Pudding 24
Pumpkin Steel-Cut Oats 24
Breakfast Scramble 25
Crazy Quinoa Protein Muffins 25
English Muffin Breakfast Sandwich 26
Mashed Chickpea Sandwich 26
Fruit and Spice Breakfast Bars 27
Quinoa Breakfast Bowls 27

Chapter 5
Snack Sensations 28
Bell Pepper Rings 29
Kale Chips 29
Apple Crisp 30
Sweet and Salty Chocolate Bark 30
Orange Cranberry Power Cookies 31
Baked Tortilla Chips 31
Cajun Spiced Pecans 32
Cherry Pecan Granola Bars 32
Mixed Berry Cobbler 33
Peanut Butter Snack Squares 33

Chapter 6
Burgers, Patties and Savory Cakes 34
Chickpea Burgers 35
Dundee Cake 36
Country Potato Patties 36
Cornmeal Cake 37
The Best Veggie Burgers 37
Depression Era Cupcakes 38
Sloppy Cajun Burgers 39
Seitan Sloppy Joes 39

Chapter 7
Rice, Grains, Potatoes Perfected 40
Broccoli-Rice Casserole 41
Breakfast Potatoes 41
Garden Pasta Salad 42
Mushroom Risotto 43
Potato Salad 43
White Bean Veggie Wrap 44
Zucchini Bread 44

Chapter 8
Soups, Stews, and Chilis 45
Split Pea Soup 46
Bean and Mushroom Chili 46
Roasted Veggie Soup 47
Sweet Squash Soup 47
Kale White Bean Soup 48
Pumpkin and Anasazi Bean Stew 49
Extra-Spicy Lentil Chili 49

Chapter 9
Meal Helpers, Veggie Sides, Dips 50
Rosemary and Thyme Brussels Sprouts 51
Thai Cabbage Salad 51
Italian Farro Salad 52
Sesame Celery Bowl 52
Tempeh Chickpea Stuffed Mini Peppers 53
Cucumber Dip 53
Corn Salad 54
Smashed Beans 54
Golden Spicy Cauliflower 55
Tomato, Corn and Bean Salad 55

Chapter 10
Divine Desserts and Drinks 56
Mini Berry Tarts 57
Salted Caramel Bites 58
Lemon Curd 58
Cinnamon Twists 59
English Muffin Protein Triangles 60
Blueberry Crisp 60
Summer Sangria 61
Vanilla Steamer 61

Appendix 1 Measurement Conversion Chart 62
Appendix 2 The Dirty Dozen and Clean Fifteen 63
Appendix 3 Index 64

Introduction

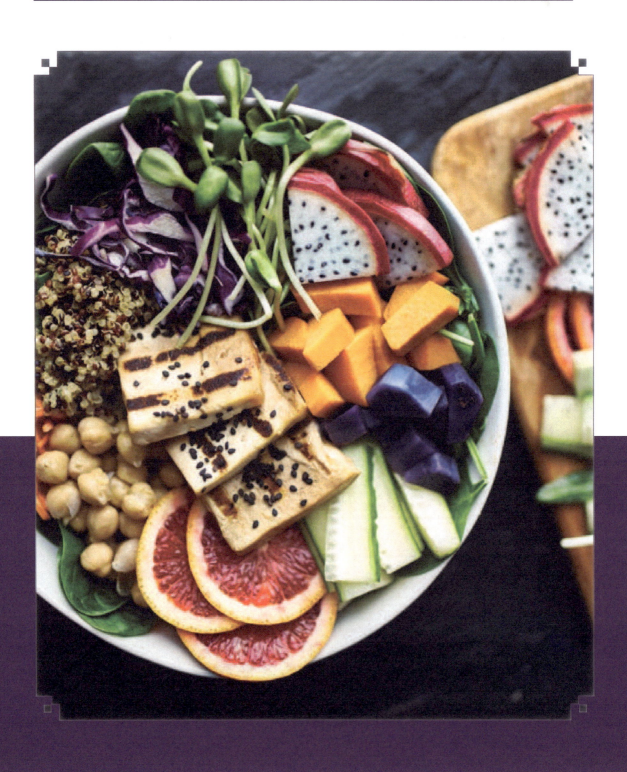

In recent years, we've witnessed a remarkable surge in the adoption of veganism as a lifestyle choice, resonating with individuals seeking a harmonious balance between personal health, compassion for animals, and environmental sustainability. As the world embraces the principles of conscious living, the demand for resources that support and inspire this journey has grown exponentially. with this in mind, I am thrilled to present to you a comprehensive guide to veganism, offering insights, recipes, and encouragement for those embarking on this transformative path.

The decision to adopt a vegan lifestyle is multifaceted, often stemming from a desire to align one's actions with values of kindness, sustainability, and optimal health. By choosing plant-based foods over animal products, we contribute to the reduction of our carbon footprint, mitigate animal suffering, and pave the way for a healthier future for ourselves and the planet we call home.

In this guide, you'll embark on a culinary journey that transcends the confines of traditional cooking. From vibrant salads bursting with seasonal produce to hearty comfort foods that evoke nostalgia without compromising on taste or ethics, each recipe is thoughtfully crafted to showcase the versatility and abundance of plant-based ingredients.

But this guide is more than just a collection of delicious recipes; it's a testament to the transformative power of food. It's about redefining our relationship with what we eat, recognizing that every meal is an opportunity to make a positive impact on our bodies, our communities, and the world around us.

As you explore the pages of this guide, you'll discover mouthwatering dishes that challenge the notion that vegan food is bland or restrictive. Instead, you'll be inspired by bold flavors, innovative techniques, and a newfound appreciation for the beauty and complexity of plant-based cuisine.

Whether you're craving a quick and satisfying weeknight meal, planning a festive gathering with loved ones, or simply seeking culinary inspiration, this guide has something for everyone. So, grab your apron, sharpen your knives, and join me on this culinary adventure as we explore the endless possibilities of vegan cooking together.

Here's to nourishing our bodies, uplifting our spirits, and creating a more compassionate world—one delicious meal at a time.

Welcome to the journey of veganism.

Chapter 1

Celebrating Your Vegan Journey

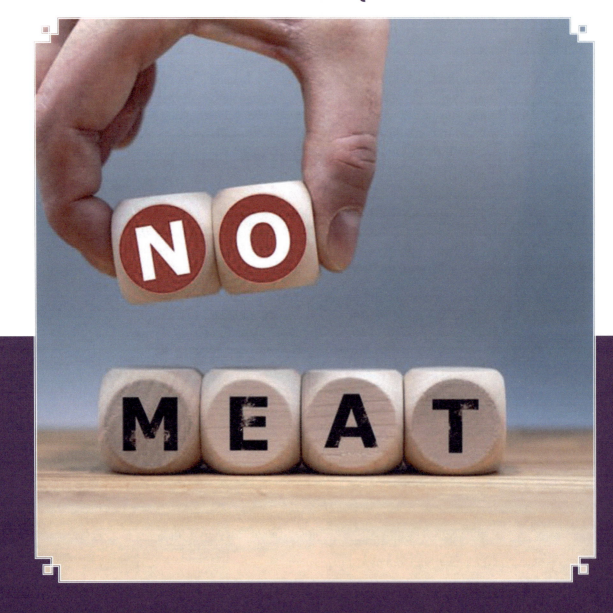

Principles and Benefits of Veganism

Veganism is more than just a dietary choice; it's a lifestyle guided by a set of principles aimed at minimizing harm to animals, protecting the environment, and promoting personal health and well-being. Understanding the core principles of veganism is essential for anyone considering or already committed to this way of life.

COMPASSION FOR ANIMALS

At the heart of veganism lies a deep sense of compassion for all living beings. Vegans choose to abstain from consuming animal products, such as meat, dairy, eggs, and honey, as well as avoiding products derived from animals, such as leather, wool, and silk. This principle extends beyond food choices to encompass all aspects of daily life, including clothing, cosmetics, and entertainment. By embracing a vegan lifestyle, individuals demonstrate their commitment to treating animals with kindness and respect, recognizing their inherent worth and right to live free from exploitation.

ENVIRONMENTAL SUSTAINABILITY

Veganism also aligns with principles of environmental sustainability, as plant-based diets have been shown to have a significantly lower environmental impact compared to diets rich in animal products. The production of meat, dairy, and eggs requires vast amounts of land, water, and resources, contributing to deforestation, water pollution, and greenhouse gas emissions. By choosing plant-based foods, vegans help reduce their ecological footprint and support more sustainable food systems. Additionally, opting for locally sourced, organic produce further minimizes environmental impact and promotes biodiversity.

HEALTH AND WELL-BEING

A well-planned vegan diet can provide all the nutrients needed for optimal health and well-being. Plant-based foods are rich in vitamins, minerals, fiber, and phytonutrients, which support immune function, improve heart health, and reduce the risk of chronic diseases such as diabetes, obesity, and certain cancers. To ensure nutritional adequacy, vegans should focus on consuming a diverse array of whole foods, including fruits, vegetables, grains, legumes, nuts, and seeds. It's also important to pay attention to nutrients that may require special consideration on a vegan diet, such as vitamin B12, vitamin D, omega-3 fatty acids, iron, and calcium, and consider supplementation or fortified foods as needed.

ADVOCACY AND EDUCATION

Vegans play a crucial role as advocates for positive change in society. By living according to their principles and sharing their experiences with others, vegans help raise awareness about the ethical, environmental, and health implications of animal agriculture. Engaging in conversations, participating in peaceful protests, and supporting animal rights organizations are just a few ways vegans can amplify their voices and inspire others to consider adopting a vegan lifestyle. Education is key to dispelling myths and misconceptions surrounding veganism and empowering individuals to make informed choices that align with their values.

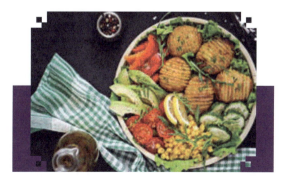

Stocking Your Vegan Kitchen

Creating a well-stocked vegan kitchen is the foundation for preparing delicious, nutritious meals that nourish the body and satisfy the palate. Whether you're a seasoned vegan or just starting out on your plant-based journey, having the right ingredients and tools on hand can make cooking easier, more enjoyable, and more fulfilling. In this guide, we'll explore five essential categories for stocking your vegan kitchen: grains and legumes, nuts and seeds, plant-based proteins, herbs and spices, and essential kitchen tools.

GRAINS AND LEGUMES

Grains and legumes serve as the backbone of many vegan meals, providing a rich source of complex carbohydrates, fiber, protein, and essential nutrients. Stock your pantry with a variety of grains such as quinoa, brown rice, barley, oats, and farro, as well as legumes like lentils, chickpeas, black beans, and kidney beans. These versatile ingredients can be used as the base for hearty salads, soups, stews, stir-fries, and grain bowls, offering endless possibilities for creating satisfying and nutritious meals.

- Practical Tip: Purchase grains and legumes in bulk to save money and reduce packaging waste, and store them in airtight containers in a cool, dry pantry or cupboard.

NUTS AND SEEDS

Nuts and seeds are nutritional powerhouses, packed with healthy fats, protein, vitamins, minerals, and antioxidants. Keep a variety of nuts such as almonds, walnuts, cashews, and peanuts, as well as seeds like chia seeds, flaxseeds, pumpkin seeds, and sunflower seeds, on hand for adding crunch, flavor, and nutrition to meals and snacks. Use nuts and seeds to make homemade nut butters, dairy-free cheeses, granolas, energy bars, and salad toppings, or enjoy them as a satisfying snack on their own.

- Practical Tip: Store nuts and seeds in the refrigerator or freezer to extend their shelf life and prevent them from going rancid due to their high oil content.

HERBS AND SPICES

Herbs and spices are the secret ingredients that elevate vegan dishes from ordinary to extraordinary, adding depth, complexity, and flavor to every bite. Keep a well-stocked spice rack or drawer with essentials like garlic powder, onion powder, cumin, paprika, chili powder, turmeric, cinnamon, ginger, oregano, basil, thyme, rosemary, and parsley, as well as fresh herbs like cilantro, basil, mint, and parsley. Use herbs and spices to season and enhance soups, sauces, marinades, dressings, dips, grains, vegetables, and proteins, allowing you to create vibrant and aromatic dishes that delight the senses.

- Practical Tip: Experiment with different flavor combinations and seasoning techniques to develop your culinary skills and customize recipes to suit your taste preferences.

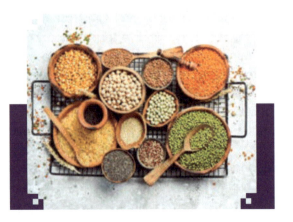

PLANT-BASED PROTEINS

Plant-based proteins are essential for building and repairing tissues, supporting immune function, and maintaining overall health and vitality. Incorporate a variety of protein-rich foods into your diet, including tofu, tempeh, seitan, edamame, soy milk, plant-based protein powders, and meat alternatives made from soy, wheat, peas, or lentils. These versatile ingredients can be used to create meatless burgers, sandwiches, tacos, stir-fries, scrambles, and more, providing satisfying and satiating meals without the need for animal products.

- Practical Tip: Experiment with different types of plant-based proteins to discover your favorites and incorporate them into your weekly meal plans for variety and balance.

ESSENTIAL KITCHEN TOOLS

Having the right kitchen tools and equipment can streamline meal preparation and make cooking more efficient and enjoyable. Invest in high-quality kitchen essentials such as sharp knives, cutting boards, mixing bowls, measuring cups and spoons, pots and pans, a blender or food processor, a vegetable peeler, a grater, a colander, a can opener, and a variety of cooking utensils. These tools will enable you to chop, slice, dice, blend, sauté, simmer, bake, and roast with ease, allowing you to unleash your creativity in the kitchen and bring your culinary creations to life.

- Practical Tip: Prioritize investing in durable, multipurpose kitchen tools that will withstand frequent use and last for years to come, and regularly maintain and sharpen knives to ensure safety and precision when cutting and slicing ingredients.

Q&As for Beginners

Q: What about essential nutrients like vitamin B12 and iron?

A: While it's true that some nutrients are more commonly found in animal products, they can still be obtained from plant-based sources or supplements. For example, vitamin B12 can be found in fortified foods such as plant-based milk, breakfast cereals, and nutritional yeast, or taken as a supplement. Iron-rich plant foods include lentils, spinach, tofu, pumpkin seeds, and fortified cereals.

Q: Will I miss out on any flavors or culinary experiences by going vegan?

A: Not at all! Vegan cuisine is incredibly diverse and flavorful, offering a wide range of delicious dishes from around the world. with a little creativity and experimentation, you can enjoy vegan versions of your favorite comfort foods, ethnic cuisines, and sweet treats, all without sacrificing taste or satisfaction.

Q: How can I deal with social situations and dining out as a vegan?

A: Dining out and navigating social situations as a vegan may require a bit of planning and communication, but it's entirely manageable. Many restaurants now offer vegan options or are willing to accommodate dietary restrictions upon request. You can also suggest vegan-friendly restaurants or offer to bring a dish to social gatherings to ensure there's something for you to eat.

Q: Will I need to spend more money on groceries as a vegan?

A: Not necessarily. While some specialty vegan products may be more expensive, many staples of a plant-based diet, such as grains, legumes, fruits, and vegetables, are affordable and widely available. Cooking meals at home using whole, unprocessed ingredients can also be cost-effective compared to dining out or buying pre-packaged foods.

Q: What advice do you have for someone just starting out on their vegan journey?

A: My advice for beginners is to start gradually and focus on making small, sustainable changes. Experiment with new recipes, explore different plant-based foods, and don't be too hard on yourself if you slip up occasionally. Surround yourself with supportive friends, family, and online communities, and remember that every vegan meal you eat makes a positive difference for animals, the environment, and your health.

Q: Will I need to take supplements on a vegan diet?

A: While a well-planned vegan diet can provide most essential nutrients, there are a few nutrients that may require special attention. One of the most important is vitamin B12, which is primarily found in animal products. Vegans should consider taking a vitamin B12 supplement or consuming fortified foods regularly. Additionally, some individuals may benefit from supplements for vitamin D, omega-3 fatty acids, iron, and calcium, depending on their individual needs and dietary intake.

Q: How can I ensure that I'm eating a balanced vegan diet?

A: Eating a balanced vegan diet involves consuming a variety of plant-based foods to meet your nutritional needs. Aim to include a variety of fruits, vegetables, whole grains, legumes, nuts, and seeds in your meals to ensure you're getting a wide range of vitamins, minerals, and phytonutrients. Pay attention to portion sizes and be mindful of including sources of protein, healthy fats, fiber, and essential nutrients in each meal. It can also be helpful to consult with a registered dietitian or nutritionist who specializes in plant-based nutrition to ensure you're meeting your individual dietary requirements.

In the pages ahead, you'll discover a wealth of delicious recipes that prove vegan cuisine is anything but bland or restrictive. From hearty main courses to decadent desserts, each dish is a testament to the creativity and versatility of plant-based ingredients. As you explore these recipes, may you find inspiration, joy, and fulfillment in the kitchen.

But this cookbook is more than just a collection of recipes; it's a call to action, inviting you to join the global movement towards a more compassionate and sustainable future. As you embrace the flavors and possibilities of vegan cooking, may you also embrace the values of empathy, mindfulness, and stewardship that define this lifestyle.

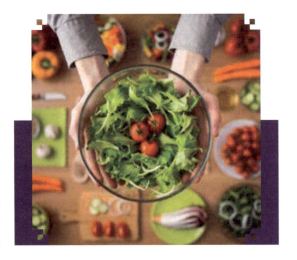

Chapter 2

4-Week Meal Plan

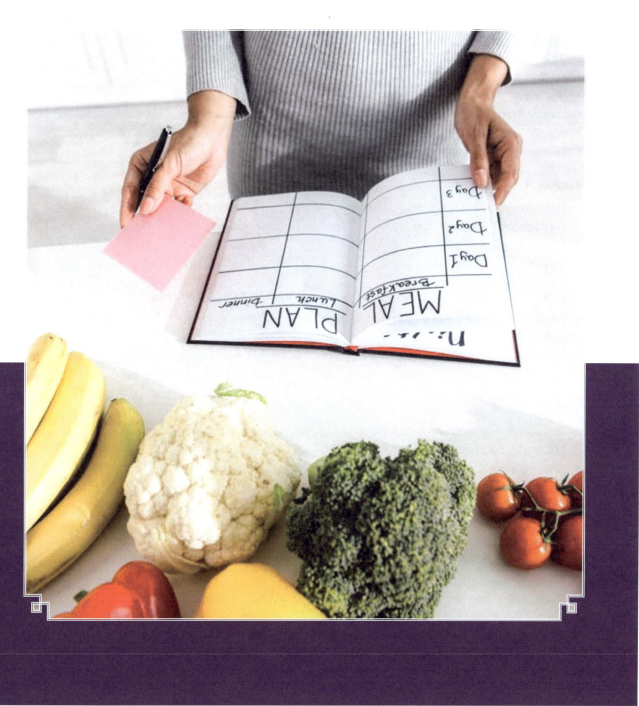

Week 1

DAY 1:
- Breakfast: Apple Oats for Breakfast
- Lunch: Black Beans Burger
- Snack: Apple Crisp
- Dinner: Rice and Noodle Pilaf

DAY 2:
- Breakfast: Apple Oats for Breakfast
- Lunch: Black Beans Burger
- Snack: Apple Crisp
- Dinner: Rice and Noodle Pilaf

DAY 3:
- Breakfast: Apple Oats for Breakfast
- Lunch: Black Beans Burger
- Snack: Apple Crisp
- Dinner: Rice and Noodle Pilaf

DAY 4:
- Breakfast: Apple Oats for Breakfast
- Lunch: Black Beans Burger
- Snack: Apple Crisp
- Dinner: Rice and Noodle Pilaf

DAY 5:
- Breakfast: Pumpkin Steel-Cut Oats
- Lunch: Black Beans Burger
- Snack: Apple Crisp
- Dinner: Rice and Noodle Pilaf

DAY 6:
- Breakfast: Pumpkin Steel-Cut Oats
- Lunch: Spiced Brown Rice
- Snack: Apple Crisp
- Dinner: Rice and Noodle Pilaf

DAY 7:
- Breakfast: Pumpkin Steel-Cut Oats
- Lunch: Spiced Brown Rice
- Snack: Apple Crisp
- Dinner: Rice and Noodle Pilaf

SHOPPING LIST:

PROTEINS:
- 1 cup black beans
- 2 tablespoons bread crumbs

VEGETABLES:
- 1 small pumpkin or ½ cup canned pumpkin purée
- 1 bunch fresh parsley
- 1 yellow sweet pepper
- 1 small onion (optional, for burger)
- 1/4 cup sweet corn, cooked

FRUITS:
- 6 Cortland apples
- 3 cups strawberries
- 2 pounds Granny Smith apples
- 1 lemon (optional)

GRAINS & LEGUMES:
- 2 cups steel-cut oats
- 5 cups long-grain brown rice
- 1 cup whole-wheat noodles
- 2 tablespoons bread crumbs

DAIRY & ALTERNATIVES:
- 1 cup cashew milk

CANNED & PACKAGED GOODS:
- 1/2 cup canned pumpkin purée
- 1/4 cup pumpkin seeds
- Maple syrup
- Vegetable broth or water
- Ground cumin
- Dried oregano
- 1/2 cup frozen unsweetened apple juice concentrate

NUTS & DRIED FRUITS:
- 1 cup cashews
- 1/2 cup chopped apricots, dried
- 1/2 cup raisins

SPICES & CONDIMENTS:
- Coconut oil
- Brown sugar
- Salt
- Turmeric
- Ground cinnamon
- Ground nutmeg
- Whole-wheat pastry flour

Week 2

DAY 1:
- Breakfast: Fruit and Spice Breakfast Bars
- Lunch: Seitan Sloppy Joes
- Snack: Real-Deal Chocolate Chip Cookies
- Dinner: Garden Pasta Salad

DAY 2:
- Breakfast: Fruit and Spice Breakfast Bars
- Lunch: Seitan Sloppy Joes
- Snack: Real-Deal Chocolate Chip Cookies
- Dinner: Garden Pasta Salad

DAY 3:
- Breakfast: Fruit and Spice Breakfast Bars
- Lunch: Seitan Sloppy Joes
- Snack: Real-Deal Chocolate Chip Cookies
- Dinner: Garden Pasta Salad

DAY 4:
- Breakfast: Fruit and Spice Breakfast Bars
- Lunch: Seitan Sloppy Joes
- Snack: Real-Deal Chocolate Chip Cookies
- Dinner: Garden Pasta Salad

DAY 5:
- Breakfast: Fruit and Spice Breakfast Bars
- Lunch: Seitan Sloppy Joes
- Snack: Real-Deal Chocolate Chip Cookies
- Dinner: Garden Pasta Salad

DAY 6:
- Breakfast: Fruit and Spice Breakfast Bars
- Lunch: Seitan Sloppy Joes
- Snack: Real-Deal Chocolate Chip Cookies
- Dinner: Garden Pasta Salad

DAY 7:
- Breakfast: Fruit and Spice Breakfast Bars
- Lunch: Garden Pasta Salad
- Snack: Real-Deal Chocolate Chip Cookies
- Dinner: Garden Pasta Salad

SHOPPING LIST:

FRUIT:
- 1 cup chopped Medjool dates
- ½ cup chopped dried apricots
- ½ cup raisins
- 1 teaspoon orange zest
- ¾ cup applesauce
- ¾ cup Best Date Syrup Ever (or substitute with another type of syrup)

GRAINS & FLOURS:
- 1 cup whole-wheat pastry flour
- 1 cup barley flour
- 2 cups all-purpose flour
- 6 toasted whole wheat buns
- 10- to 12-ounce package tricolor rotini pasta

PROTEIN:
- 2 cups seitan

VEGETABLES:
- 1 cup chopped broccoli
- 1 cup chopped cauliflower
- 1 cup snow peas, trimmed
- 1 cup sliced mushrooms
- 3 scallions
- 2-ounce jar chopped pimientos, drained
- ¾ cup cherry tomatoes

SAUCES & CONDIMENTS:
- 8 ounces tomato sauce
- 1 tablespoon vegan Worcestershire sauce
- 2 tablespoons red wine vinegar
- ⅓ cup organic ketchup

- ¾ to 1 cup oil-free Italian dressing

BAKING ESSENTIALS:
- 1 tablespoon baking powder
- 1 teaspoon ground cinnamon
- 1 teaspoon ground ginger
- ¼ teaspoon ground cloves
- 1 teaspoon almond extract
- 1 tablespoon flaxseed meal
- 1 teaspoon vanilla extract
- 1 teaspoon baking soda

SWEETENERS:
- 1 cup brown sugar
- ½ cup granulated sugar
- ¾ cup vegan semisweet chocolate chips
- Coconut sugar (optional, for Seitan Sloppy Joes)

OTHER:
- Sea salt
- Margarine (for greasing)
- Freshly ground black pepper

Week 3

DAY 1:
- Breakfast: Easy Nonfat Garlic Bread
- Lunch: The Best Veggie Burgers
- Snack: Peanut Butter Snack Squares
- Dinner: Mushroom Risotto

DAY 2:
- Breakfast: Easy Nonfat Garlic Bread
- Lunch: The Best Veggie Burgers
- Snack: Peanut Butter Snack Squares
- Dinner: Mushroom Risotto

DAY 3:
- Breakfast: Easy Nonfat Garlic Bread
- Lunch: The Best Veggie Burgers
- Snack: Peanut Butter Snack Squares
- Dinner: Mushroom Risotto

DAY 4:
- Breakfast: Easy Nonfat Garlic Bread
- Lunch: The Best Veggie Burgers
- Snack: Peanut Butter Snack Squares
- Dinner: Mushroom Risotto

DAY 5:
- Breakfast: Easy Nonfat Garlic Bread
- Lunch: The Best Veggie Burgers
- Snack: Peanut Butter Snack Squares
- Dinner: White Bean Veggie Wrap

DAY 6:
- Breakfast: Easy Nonfat Garlic Bread
- Lunch: The Best Veggie Burgers
- Snack: Peanut Butter Snack Squares
- Dinner: White Bean Veggie Wrap

DAY 7:
- Breakfast: Easy Nonfat Garlic Bread
- Lunch: White Bean Veggie Wrap
- Snack: Peanut Butter Snack Squares
- Dinner: White Bean Veggie Wrap

SHOPPING LIST:

PROTEINS:
- ½ cup walnuts
- 2 cups precooked green lentils or brown lentils
- 1 (15-ounce) can red kidney beans
- 1 cup white beans (for white bean spread)
- ½ cup peanuts

VEGETABLES:
- 5 cloves garlic
- parsley flakes (optional)
- 1 yellow onion
- 1 red onion
- 1 red bell pepper
- 1 medium zucchini
- 1 medium yellow squash
- basil
- scallions (green parts only)

- 9 ounces baby portabella mushrooms
- 4 ounces shiitake mushrooms

SPICES & HERBS:
- Paprika
- Ground cinnamon
- Ground ginger
- Ground cloves
- Sea salt
- Vanilla extract
- Baking powder
- Tomato paste
- Vegan Worcestershire sauce
- Tamari
- Red wine vinegar
- Dijon mustard or yellow mustard

GRAINS & FLOURS:
- 1 loaf whole-wheat french bread
- 1 cup whole-wheat pastry flour
- 1 cup barley flour
- 2 1/4 cups all-purpose flour (for chocolate chip cookies)
- 1 cup precooked brown rice
- 1 1/2 cups arborio rice
- 3/4 to 1 cup coarse cornmeal
- 3/4 cup whole wheat flour
- 1/4 cup garbanzo flour
- 1 cup old-fashioned oats
- 4 12-inch whole-grain flatbreads

DAIRY & ALTERNATIVES:
- ½ cup dairy-free milk
- Margarine (for greasing)

CONDIMENTS & SAUCES:
- 1 cup oil-free Italian dressing
- 2 tablespoons tomato paste
- 1 tablespoon vegan worcestershire sauce
- 1 tablespoon tamari
- 2 tablespoons red wine vinegar
- ⅓ cup organic ketchup
- 1 tablespoon dijon mustard or yellow mustard
- 1 cup white bean spread or hummus

- 1 cup best date syrup ever
- ½ cup coconut sugar
- 1 cup brown sugar
- ½ cup granulated sugar
- 2 tablespoons maple syrup

BAKING ESSENTIALS:
- Baking powder
- Vanilla extract
- Baking soda

Week 4

DAY 1:
- Breakfast: Breakfast Scramble
- Lunch: Cornmeal Cake
- Snack: Mixed Berry Cobbler
- Dinner: Ricotta Red Sauce Pasta

DAY 2:
- Breakfast: Breakfast Scramble
- Lunch: Cornmeal Cake
- Snack: Mixed Berry Cobbler
- Dinner: Ricotta Red Sauce Pasta

DAY 3:
- Breakfast: Breakfast Scramble
- Lunch: Cornmeal Cake
- Snack: Mixed Berry Cobbler
- Dinner: Ricotta Red Sauce Pasta

DAY 4:
- Breakfast: Breakfast Scramble
- Lunch: Cornmeal Cake
- Snack: Mixed Berry Cobbler
- Dinner: Ricotta Red Sauce Pasta

DAY 5:
- Breakfast: Breakfast Scramble
- Lunch: Cornmeal Cake
- Snack: Mixed Berry Cobbler
- Dinner: Spiced Brown Rice

DAY 6:
- Breakfast: Spring Breakfast Salad
- Lunch: Cornmeal Cake
- Snack: Mixed Berry Cobbler
- Dinner: Spiced Brown Rice

DAY 7:
- Breakfast: Spring Breakfast Salad
- Lunch: Cornmeal Cake
- Snack: Mixed Berry Cobbler
- Dinner: Spiced Brown Rice

SHOPPING LIST:

VEGETABLES:
- 1 medium red onion
- 1 medium red bell pepper
- 1 medium green bell pepper
- 2 cups sliced mushrooms
- 1 large head cauliflower (or two 19-ounce cans Jamaican ackee)
- ¼ cup chopped fresh mint

FRUITS:
- ½ cup strawberries
- ½ cup blueberries
- ½ cup blackberries
- ½ cup raspberries
- 1 grapefruit
- 1 orange

DAIRY & ALTERNATIVES:
- 1 cup cashews (for soaking)
- 1 block firm tofu
- Vegan butter
- 1 cup plant-based milk

GRAINS & FLOURS:
- 1½ cups coarse cornmeal or polenta
- 10 ounces chickpea-based pasta
- 1 1/2 cups brown rice
- 1 cup whole wheat or all-purpose flour

NUTS & SEEDS:
- 1/4 cup sliced almonds
- 1/2 cup cashews
- 1/2 cup roasted cashews

CANNED GOODS:
- Two 19-ounce cans Jamaican ackee (if not using cauliflower)

CONDIMENTS & SAUCES:
- 1 to 2 tablespoons low-sodium soy sauce
- 1 1/2 cups vegan red pasta sauce
- Canola or vegetable oil

BAKING ESSENTIALS:
- Baking powder

SPICES & HERBS:
- Salt
- Freshly ground black pepper
- 1½ teaspoons turmeric
- ¼ teaspoon cayenne pepper
- 3 cloves garlic
- 1½ tablespoons B12-fortified nutritional yeast
- 1 teaspoon dried oregano
- ½ teaspoon dried basil

SWEETENERS:
- 1 tablespoon pure maple syrup
- ⅔ cup granulated sugar

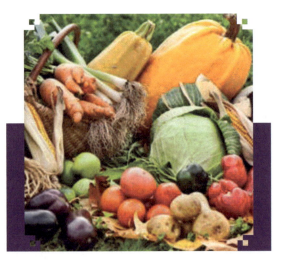

Chapter 3

Versatile Sauces and Fillings

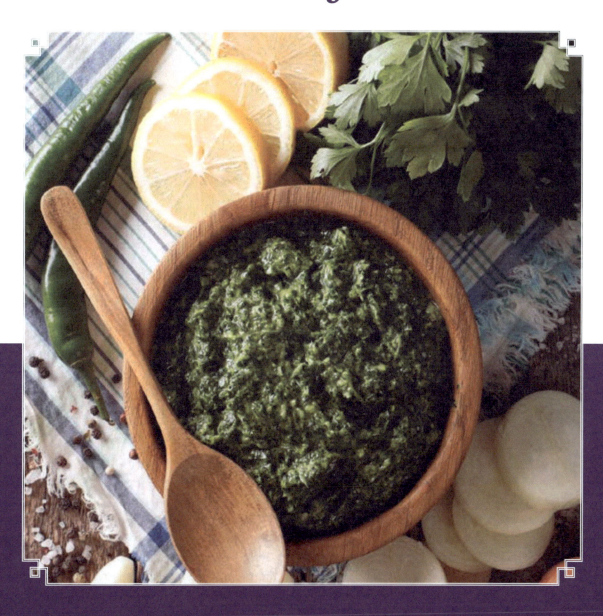

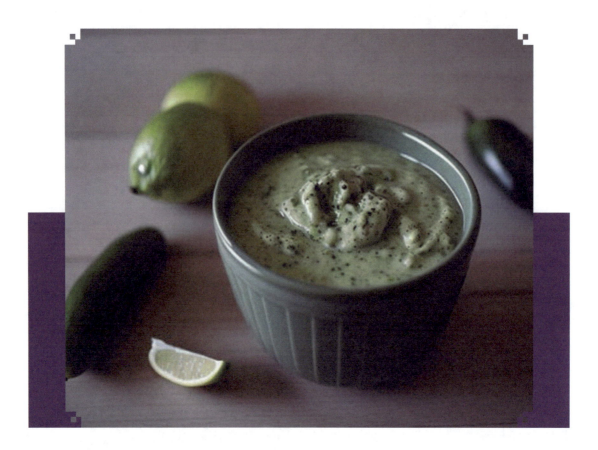

Mexican Rice Filling

Prep time: 10 minutes | Cooking time: 4 minutes | Servings: 6

- ½ cup black beans, canned
- 2 cups of water
- 1 cup of rice
- 1 tsp salt
- 1 tbsp olive oil
- ½ tsp paprika
- 1 tsp chili flakes

1. Place rice and water in the instant pot. Add salt and corn kernels.
2. When the rice and corn are cooked, chill them to the room temperature and add in the bean's mixture. Mix up well.

Cucumber Dressing

Prep time: 5 minutes | Cook time: 5 minutes | Serves 2

- 1 cup cooked white beans
- ¼ cup fresh lemon juice
- zest of 1 lemon
- 2 large cucumbers, peeled, seeded, and coarsely chopped
- 1 clove garlic
- sea salt to taste
- pinch of cayenne pepper

1. Combine all ingredients in a blender and purée until smooth and creamy.
2. Store refrigerated in an airtight container for up to seven days.

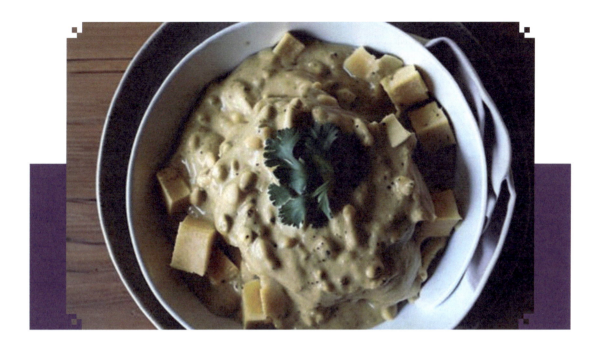

Cheesy Vegetable Sauce

Prep time: 10 minutes | Cook time: 25 minutes | Serves 4

- 1 cup raw cashews
- 1 russet potato, peeled and cubed
- 2 carrots, cubed
- ½ cup nutritional yeast
- 1 onion, chopped
- 3 garlic cloves, minced
- 1 tablespoon water, plus more as needed

1. In an 8-quart pot, combine the cashews, potato, and carrots. Add enough water to cover by 2 inches. Bring to a boil over high heat, then reduce the heat to simmer. Cook for 15 minutes.
2. In a blender, combine the nutritional yeast, miso paste, ground mustard, milk, and arrowroot powder.
3. Use immediately, or refrigerate in a sealable container for up to 1 week.

Caesar-Style Dressing

Prep time: 5 minutes | Cook time: none | Serves 3

- 3 tablespoons vegan mayonnaise
- 2 tablespoons vegan Worcestershire sauce
- 1 tablespoon Dijon mustard
- 1 teaspoon red wine vinegar
- 4 teaspoons minced garlic (about 4 cloves)
- ¾ cup extra-virgin olive oil
- ¼ cup nutritional yeast
- ¼ teaspoon salt
- ¼ teaspoon freshly ground black pepper

1. In a blender or food processor, combine the mayonnaise, Worcestershire, mustard, vinegar, and garlic. Blend until the ingredients are well combined. You might need to stop and scrape down the sides during this process to ensure all ingredients are mixed well.
2. Transfer to a wide-mouth pint jar and close tightly with a lid.

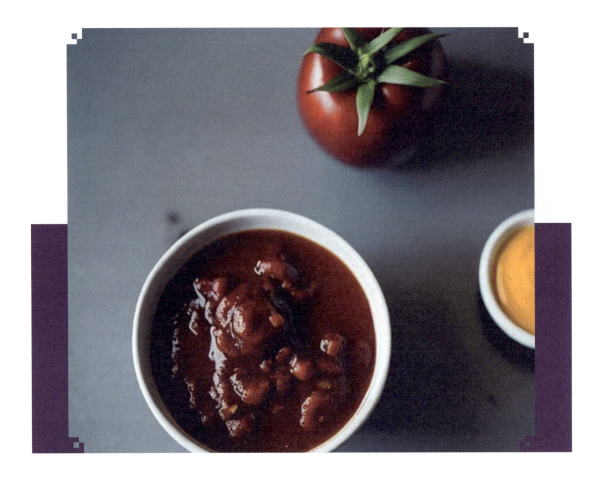

Green Enchilada Sauce

Prep time: 5 minutes | Cook time: 10 minutes | Makes 1 quart

- one 7-ounce can mexican green sauce
- 3½ cups water
- 4 tablespoons cornstarch
  chopped fresh cilantro for garnish (optional)

1. Combine all of the ingredients except the cilantro.
2. Cook over medium heat, stirring constantly, until the mixture boils and thickens. Add the cilantro just before using.

Homemade Ketchup

Prep time: 5 minutes | Cook time: 20 minutes | Serves 12

- 2 lbs. firm tomatoes, quartered
- ½ cup apple cider vinegar
- ½ teaspoon granulated garlic
- ¼ teaspoon ground clove
- ¼ cup golden raisins
- ½ teaspoon salt

1. Combine all the ingredients in the Instant Pot and stir.
2. If desired, pass the ketchup through a sieve to remove small lumps.

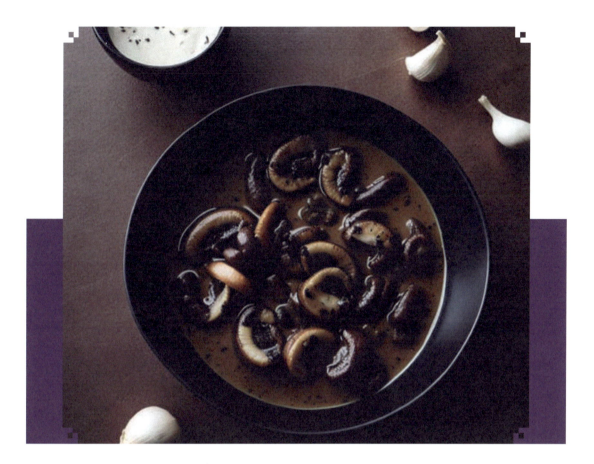

Mango Salad Dressing

Prep time: 5 minutes | Cook time: 5 minutes | Serves 3

- 2 large mangoes, peeled, seeded, and coarsely chopped
- ½ cup fresh orange juice
- ½ cup rice wine vinegar
- ¼ cup brown rice syrup
- ¼ teaspoon sea salt
- ¼ teaspoon crushed red pepper

1. Combine all ingredients in a blender and purée until smooth and creamy.
2. Store refrigerated in an airtight container for up to seven days.

Garlic-Mushroom Sauce

Prep time: 10 minutes | Cook time: 6 minutes | Makes 2 cups

- 1 cup sliced mushrooms
- 2 tablespoons soy sauce
- 1 clove garlic, pressed
- 1 teaspoon grated fresh ginger

1. Place the mushrooms in a saucepan with 1⁄4 cup of the water. Sauté until the mushrooms are softened slightly, about 4 minutes.
2. Add the remaining 11⁄2 cups water and the cornstarch mixture. Season with the pepper and sesame oil.

From Garden to Table | 17

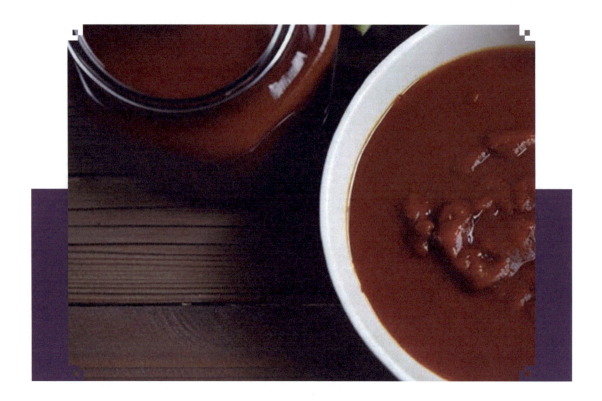

Creamy Leek Sauce

Prep time: 5 minutes | Cook time: 15 minutes | Serves 2½

- 2 large leeks, thinly sliced
- 1½ teaspoon thyme, minced
- pinch of ground nutmeg
- 2 cups cauliflower purée
- Sea salt and black pepper to taste

1. In a large saucepan, sauté the leeks over medium heat for 7 to 8 minutes.
2. Add water 1 to 2 tablespoons at a time to keep the leeks from sticking.
3. Add the thyme and nutmeg and cook for 1 minute.
4. Add the cauliflower purée and cook over medium-low heat for 5 minutes.
5. Season with salt and pepper.

Mild Harissa Sauce

Prep time: 10 minutes | Cook time: 20 minutes | Serves 3 to 4

- 1 large red bell pepper, seeded, cored, and cut into chunks
- 1 yellow onion, cut into thick rings
- 4 garlic cloves, peeled
- 1 tablespoon Hungarian paprika
- 1 teaspoon ground cumin

1. Preheat the oven to 450°F. Line a baking sheet with parchment paper or aluminum foil.
2. Place the bell pepper on the prepared baking sheet, flesh-side up, and space out the onion and garlic around the pepper.
3. Refrigerate in an airtight container for up to 2 weeks or freeze for up to 6 months.

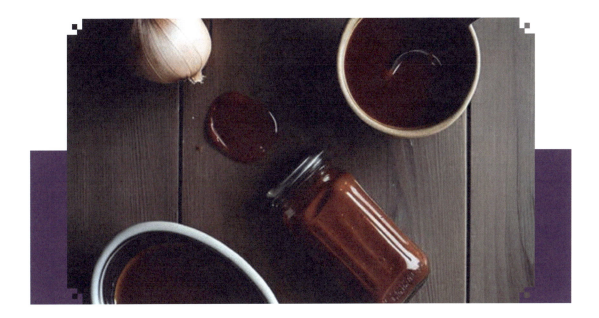

Yellow Pepper Sauce

Prep time: 20 minutes | **Cook time:** 35 minutes | Serves 6 to 8

- 4 medium yellow bell peppers
- 2 medium potatoes
- 1 cup water
- 2 tablespoons white wine
- 1 tablespoon fresh lemon juice
- 1½ teaspoons soy sauce
- 1 teaspoon onion powder
- ¼ teaspoon freshly ground white pepper

1. Clean and chop the peppers and peel and chop the potatoes. Place in a saucepan with the water. Cover and cook over low heat for 30 minutes. Remove from the heat. Pour into a blender or food processor.
2. Blend until smooth. Return to the saucepan and add the remaining ingredients. Heat through to allow the flavors to blend.

Buffalo-Style Barbecue Sauce

Prep time: 10 minutes | **Cook time:** 25 minutes | Serves 2

- 1 tablespoon vegetable oil or extra-virgin olive oil
- ½ cup chopped onion
- 1 teaspoon minced garlic (about 1 clove)
- 1 cup ketchup
- ½ cup hot sauce
- ¼ cup apple cider vinegar
- 1 tablespoon vegan Worcestershire sauce
- salt

1. In a medium saucepan over medium-low heat, heat the vegetable oil. Add the onion and garlic and cook for 5 minutes, stirring, until softened. Reduce the heat to low.
2. Pour into a mason jar or airtight container. Let cool before sealing the lid.

Chapter 4

Breakfast and Brunch Creations

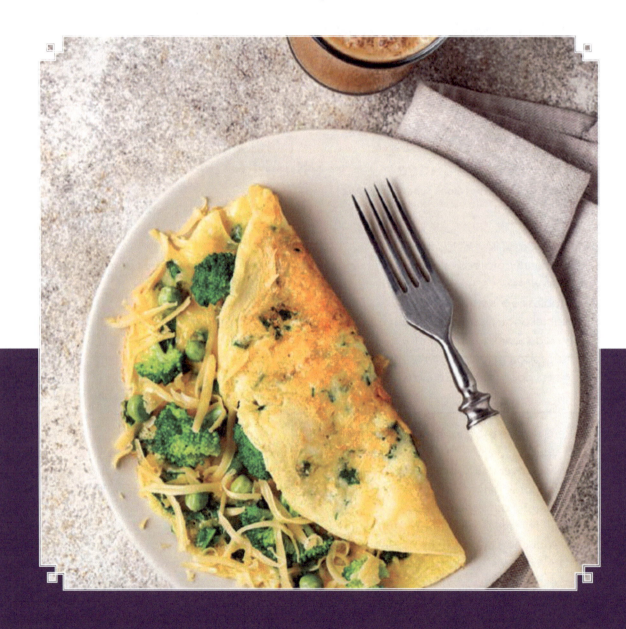

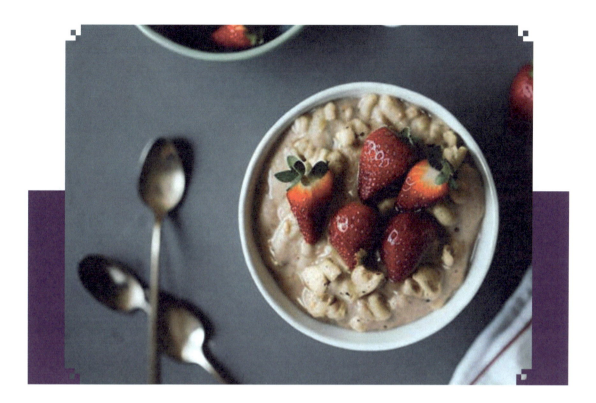

Strawberry Oatmeal

Prep time: 5 minutes| Cook time: 3 minutes | Serves 4

- 2 cups rolled oats
- 1 handful chopped strawberries
- 4 cups water
- 1 tbsp maple syrup
- 2 tbsp flax meal

1. Combine all the fixings in the Instant Pot. Stir well.
2. Secure the lid and start the cooker using the manual setting for 3 minutes on high.
3. Natural release the pressure for about 10 minutes. Quick release and serve.
4. Portion into the dishes and top with a few berries. Relax and enjoy.

Apple Oats for Breakfast

Prep time: 10 minutes| Cook time: 20 minutes| Serves 4

- ½ cup steel-cut oats
- 3 cups, water
- 1 tbsp brown sugar
- 1 pinch salt
- 1 cup cashew milk
- 1 cup fresh halved strawberries

1. Grease the Instant Pot with the oil and add the fixings – except for the berries and milk.
2. Securely lock the lid and set the timer for ten minutes using the high-pressure setting.
3. Adjust to your taste and serve with a portion of strawberries and milk.

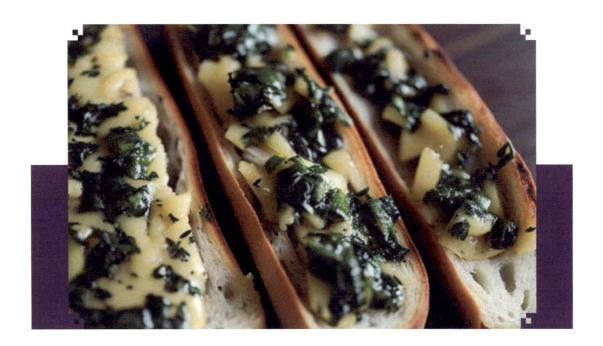

Sweet Potato Toast

Prep time: 5 minutes | Cook time: 6 minutes | Makes 6–8 slices

- 1 small sweet potato
- oil for misting
- date paste
- 1–2 tablespoons grated coconut
- sliced almonds and dried cranberries for topping

1. Preheat the air fryer to 390°F.
2. Cut the sweet potato into slices between 1/4-inch and 1/2-inch thick.
3. Spray one side of the sweet potato slices with oil.
4. Flip them over and spread a layer of Date Paste to taste on the other side.
5. Before serving, top the sweet potatoes with sliced almonds and dried cranberries, or sprinkle them with the spices or toppings of your choice.

Easy Nonfat Garlic Bread

Prep time: 15 minutes | Cook time: 5 minutes | Serves 12

- 1 cup oil-free Italian dressing
- 1 teaspoon paprika
- 5 cloves garlic (or more to taste)
- 1 loaf whole-wheat french bread
- parsley flakes (optional)

1. Preheat the broiler.
2. Place the dressing, paprika, and garlic in a blender and process until well blended. Brush this mixture on the bread and sprinkle with parsley, if desired.
3. Broil until the bread turns a light golden brown. Watch carefully to make sure it doesn't burn.
4. Note: The garlic mixture will stay fresh for several weeks in the refrigerator if stored in a covered container.

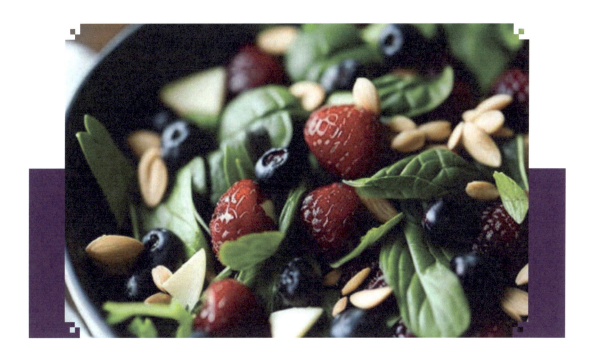

Cinnamon Donut Bites

Prep time: 10 minutes | Cook time: 6 minutes | Serves 4

- 2 tbsp ground flaxseed
- 6 tbsp water
- 1 cup plus 2 tbsp all-purpose flour
- ½ tsp kosher salt
- 2 tsp ground cinnamon, divided
- ¼ cup light brown sugar
- ¼ cup unsweetened soy milk
- 1 tbsp melted coconut oil
- ¼ cup granulated sugar

1. In a small bowl, combine the flaxseed and water. Mix well.
2. Place the balls in the fryer basket and cook until puffed and golden brown, about 6 minutes.
3. Transfer the donut bites to a platter and serve immediately.

Spring Breakfast Salad

Prep time: 10 minutes | Cook time: 15 minutes | Serves 2

- ½ cup strawberries
- ½ cup blueberries
- ½ cup blackberries
- ½ cup raspberries
- 1 grapefruit, peeled and segmented
- 3 tablespoons fresh orange juice (from 1 orange)
- 1 tablespoon pure maple syrup
- ¼ cup chopped fresh mint
- ¼ cup sliced almonds

1. In a serving bowl, combine the berries and grapefruit.
2. In a small bowl, stir together the orange juice and maple syrup. Pour the syrup mixture over the fruit. Sprinkle with the mint and almonds. Serve immediately.

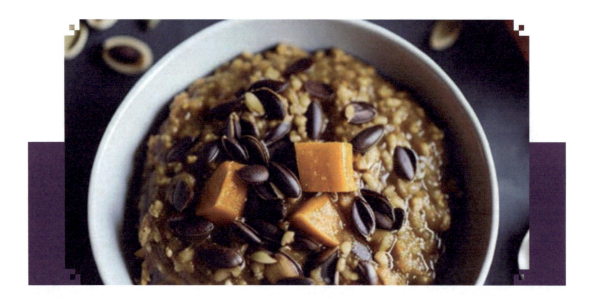

Strawberry-Kiwi Chia Pudding

Prep time: 5 minutes, plus 4 hours | **Cook time:** 15 minutes | **Serves 2**

- 2 cups unsweetened coconut milk, divided
- 3 medjool dates, pitted
- 1 tablespoon vanilla extract
- ½ cup chia seeds

Toppings:
- 2 kiwis, sliced
- 4 strawberries, sliced
- 2 tablespoons sliced or chopped almonds

1. In a food processor, blend ¾ cup of coconut milk, the dates, and vanilla.
2. Store in the refrigerator overnight or for at least 4 hours, until the chia seeds absorb all the milk. (Optional: stir once or twice as it is setting to avoid clumps.)
3. When ready to eat, top the pudding with the kiwi, strawberries, coconut, and almonds.
4. Store in the refrigerator for up to 5 days.

Pumpkin Steel-Cut Oats

Prep time: 2 minutes | **Cook time:** 35 minutes | **Serves 4**

- 3 cups water
- 1 cup steel-cut oats
- ½ cup canned pumpkin purée
- ¼ cup pumpkin seeds
- 2 tablespoons maple syrup
- pinch salt

1. In a large saucepan, bring the water to a boil.
2. Add the oats, stir, and reduce the heat to low. Simmer until the oats are soft, 20 to 30 minutes, continuing to stir occasionally.
3. Stir in the pumpkin purée and continue cooking on low for 3 to 5 minutes longer. Stir in the pumpkin seeds and maple syrup, and season with the salt.
4. Divide the oatmeal into 4 single-serving containers. Let cool before sealing the lids.

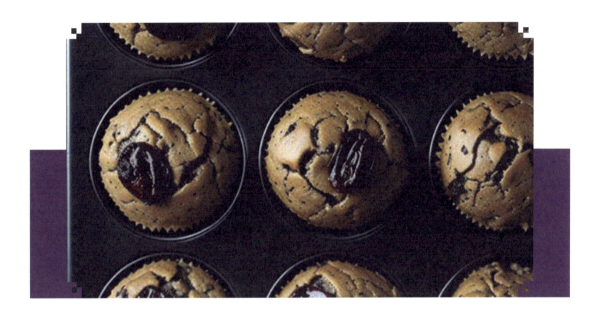

Breakfast Scramble

Prep time: 10 minutes | Cook time: 15 minutes | Serves 6

- 1 medium red onion, peeled and cut into ½-inch dice
- 1 medium red bell pepper, seeded and cut into ½-inch dice
- ¼ teaspoon cayenne pepper, or to taste
- 3 cloves garlic, peeled and minced
- 1 to 2 tablespoons low-sodium soy sauce
- ¼ cup nutritional yeast, optional

1. Place the onion, red and green peppers, and mushrooms in a medium skillet or saucepan and sauté over medium-high heat for 7 to 8 minutes, or until the onion is translucent.
2. Add the salt, black pepper, turmeric, cayenne pepper, garlic, soy sauce, and nutritional yeast (if using) to the pan and cook for 5 minutes more, or until hot and fragrant.

Crazy Quinoa Protein Muffins

Prep time: 20 minutes | Cook time: 35 minutes | Serves 6

- ½ cup quinoa
- 3 tablespoons vanilla protein powder
- ½ teaspoon salt
- ½ cup dates, chopped small
- 2 tablespoons coconut oil
- 3 tablespoons maple syrup
- 1 teaspoon vanilla extract
- ½ cup raisins

1. Rinse the quinoa and place in a small saucepan with a lid. Take off the lid and let cool.
2. Preheat the oven to 450°F. Line six muffin cups with paper liners.
3. Divide the batter between the six muffin cups and bake 12 to 15 minutes, until a toothpick inserted in the center comes out clean.

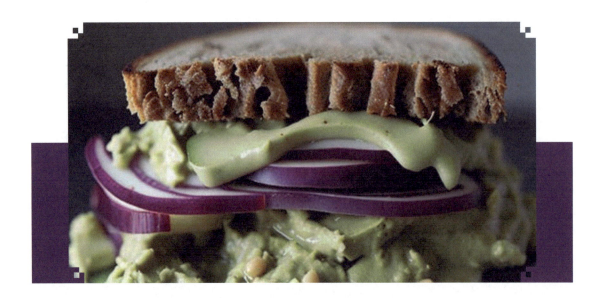

English Muffin Breakfast Sandwich

Prep time: 15 minutes | Cook time: 5 minutes | Serves 4

- 1 medium red apple
- 4 whole English muffins
- 3/4 cup Cheddar-style shreds
- ground cinnamon
- 1/4 cup coarsely chopped walnuts
- 1/4 cup dried cranberries

1. Preheat the air fryer to 390°F.
2. Quarter and core the apple and cut each quarter lengthwise into 1/4-inch slices.
3. Split 2 of the English muffins and lay them cut-side up.
4. Transfer to a plate. Close each muffin and use a spatula to press the tops down firmly.
5. While the first batch is cooking, repeat above steps to assemble remaining muffins. Cook as above and serve hot.

Mashed Chickpea Sandwich

Prep time: 10 minutes | Cook time: none | Serves 4

- 1 large ripe avocado, halved and pitted
- 1 (15-ounce) can chickpeas, drained and rinsed
- 1/4 cup diced red onion
- 1 celery stalk, diced
- 1 teaspoon Dijon mustard
- 1 teaspoon dried dill
- 1/2 teaspoon garlic powder

1. Scoop the avocado flesh into a medium bowl. Using a potato masher or a heavy spoon, mash the avocado until smooth.
2. Add the chickpeas and mash lightly so some larger pieces of chickpea remain for texture.
3. Using a spoon or spatula, mix in the pickle (if using), red onion, celery, mustard, dill, and garlic powder. Serve or refrigerate overnight for an even more blended flavor.

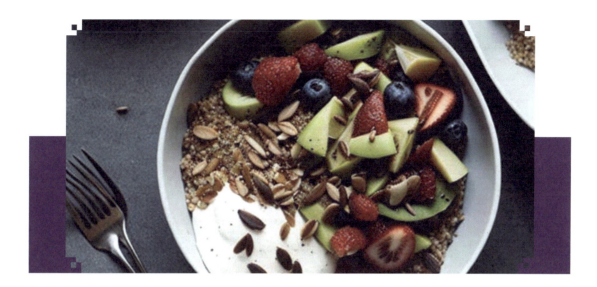

Fruit and Spice Breakfast Bars

Prep time: 5 minutes | Cook time: 5 minutes | Serves 8

- 1 cup whole-wheat pastry flour
- 1 cup barley flour
- 1 tablespoon baking powder
- 1 teaspoon ground cinnamon
- 1 teaspoon orange zest
- 1 teaspoon almond extract
- ½ cup chopped Medjool dates
- ½ cup raisins

1. Preheat the oven to 350 degrees F. Line an 8×8 inch square baking pan with parchment paper and set aside.
2. Gently fold the applesauce mixture and the dates, apricots, and raisins into the flour mixture.
3. Spread the batter in the prepared pan and bake for 30 to 35 minutes, until a toothpick inserted in the center of the pan comes out clean. Let cool before cutting into squares.

Quinoa Breakfast Bowls

Prep time: 5 minutes | Cook time: 20 minutes | Serves 4

- 1 cup quinoa, rinsed and drained
- ½ tsp pure vanilla extract
- pinch of ground cinnamon

For Serving:
- ¼ cup pure maple syrup
- 1 cup berries (any combination of blueberries, raspberries, or strawberries)
- 1 banana, sliced

1. In the inner pot, stir together the quinoa, almond milk, vanilla, and cinnamon. Lock the lid and ensure the steam release valve is set to the sealing position. Select Pressure Cook (High), and set the cook time for 5 minutes.
2. Once the cook time is complete, immediately quick release the pressure. Carefully remove the lid.
3. 3 If desired, stir in more milk to thin into a to taste with maple syrup and topped generously with fruit and almonds.

From Garden to Table

Chapter 5

Snack Sensations

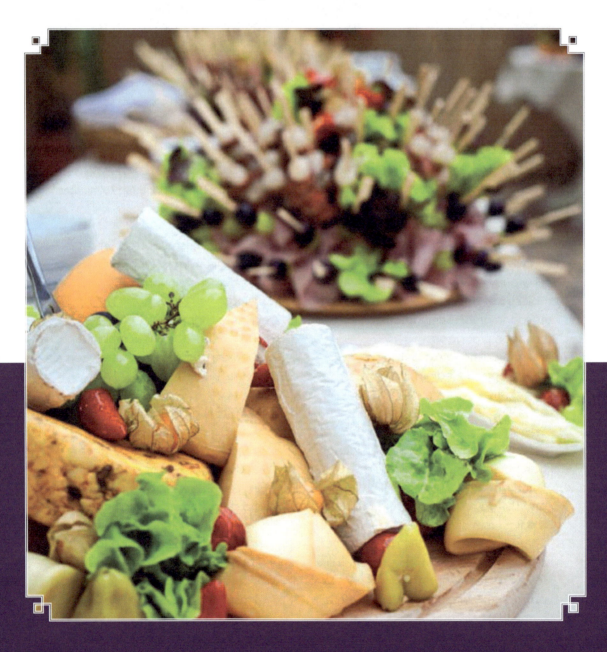

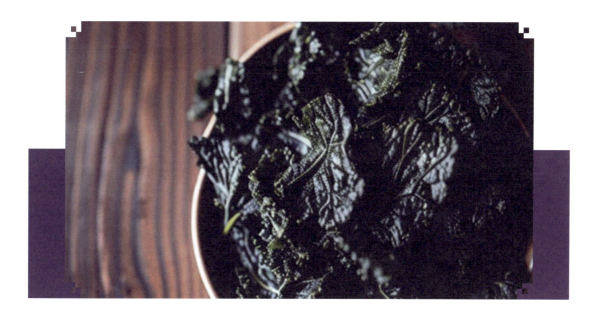

Bell Pepper Rings

Prep time: 15 minutes | **Cook time:** 14 minutes | Serves 4

- 2 large bell peppers
- 1/2 cup all-purpose white flour
- 1/2 teaspoon salt
- 1/2 cup lemon-lime soda
- 1/2 cup crushed panko breadcrumbs
- 1/2 cup plain breadcrumbs
- oil for misting or cooking spray

1. Preheat the air fryer to 390°F.
2. Slice the bell peppers widthwise into 1/4-inch rings. Remove the seeds and membranes.
3. In a large bowl, stir together the flour and salt.
4. Slowly pour the soda into the flour mixture and stir until the foaming stops and you have a medium-thick batter.
5. Cook for an additional 3 to 4 minutes, until golden brown and crispy.

Kale Chips

Prep time: 5 minutes | **Cook time:** 25 minutes | Serves 2

- 1 large bunch kale
- 1 tablespoon extra-virgin olive oil
- ½ teaspoon chipotle powder
- ½ teaspoon smoked paprika
- ¼ teaspoon salt

1. Preheat the oven to 275°F. Line a large baking sheet with parchment paper.
2. In a large bowl, stem the kale and tear it into bite-size pieces. Add the olive oil, chipotle powder, smoked paprika, and salt. Toss the kale with tongs or your hands, coating each piece well.
3. Spread the kale over the parchment paper in a single layer. Bake for 25 minutes, turning halfway through, until crisp.
4. Cool for 10 to 15 minutes before dividing and storing in 2 airtight containers.

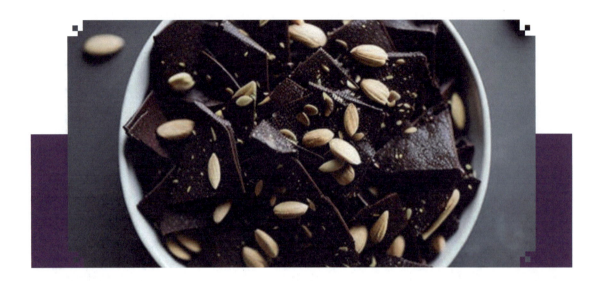

Apple Crisp

Prep time: 25 minutes | Cook time: 30 minutes | Serves 8 to 10

- 1/2 cup old-fashioned rolled oats
- 1/2 cup frozen unsweetened apple juice concentrate, thawed
- 2 pounds granny smith apples, sliced
- 1/2 teaspoon ground cinnamon
- 1/4 teaspoon ground nutmeg
- 1 tablespoon whole-wheat pastry flour

1. Preheat the oven to 425°F.
2. Coarsely chop the oats in a food processor or a blender. Stir in 1 tablespoon of the apple juice concentrate. Set aside.
3. Place the apples in a mixing bowl and mix with the remainder of the apple juice concentrate. Add the cinnamon, nutmeg, and flour. Toss to coat.
4. Place the apples in a nonstick 13 × 9-inch pan. Crumble the oat topping over the apples. Bake for 30 minutes, or until hot, bubbly, and golden brown.

Sweet and Salty Chocolate Bark

Prep time: 5 minutes | Cook time: 15 minutes | Serves 6

- 1/4 cup dried cranberries
- 3 tablespoons chopped pistachios
- 3 tablespoons chopped almonds
- 3 tablespoons sunflower seeds
- pink himalayan salt

1. Line an 8-inch square baking pan with parchment paper. Spread out the cranberries, pistachios, almonds, pumpkin seeds, and sunflower seeds on the baking pan.
2. In a small nonstick saucepan on low heat, gently heat the chocolate chips, stirring continuously, until they are melted and smooth.
3. Pour the melted chocolate evenly over the nuts, seeds, and dried fruit temperature. Sprinkle with salt. Break the bark into pieces and remove from the baking pan.

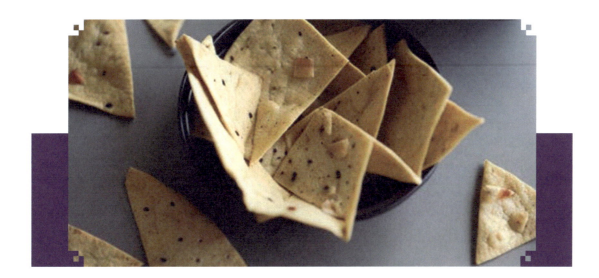

Orange Cranberry Power Cookies

Prep time: 20 minutes | Cook time: 35 minutes | Serves 12

- 1 cup dairy-free butter, softened
- 2 tablespoons protein powder
- 1 teaspoon baking powder
- ¼ teaspoon baking soda
- 1 cup old-fashioned oats
- 1 cup dairy-free chocolate chips
- 1 cup walnuts, chopped
- 1 cup dried cranberries

1. Preheat the oven to 375°F.
2. Beat the butter and sugar together in the bowl of a stand mixer. Add the orange juice and vanilla extract. Mix well.
3. Drop heaping tablespoons about 2 inches apart on an ungreased baking sheet. These are big cookies. They spread out to 3 to 4 inches in diameter. Bake for 10 to 11 minutes.
4. Cool a minute and then transfer to a wire rack to cool completely.

Baked Tortilla Chips

Prep time: 10 minutes | Cook time: 15 minutes | Serves 6

- 12 organic corn tortillas
- ¼ teaspoon chili powder
- ¼ teaspoon ground cumin
- ¼ teaspoon garlic powder
- ¼ teaspoon paprika
- 1 teaspoon organic virgin coconut oil, melted
- sea salt

1. Preheat the oven to 425°F. Line 2 baking sheets with parchment paper.
2. Cut each tortilla into 6 wedges, then arrange the wedges in an even layer on the prepared baking sheets. Bake for 10 minutes.
3. Remove from the oven and very lightly brush one side of the chips with the oil. (Too much oil and the chips will be chewy.) Sprinkle evenly with the spices and salt. Return the pans to the oven and bake for 5 to 8 minutes, or until golden.

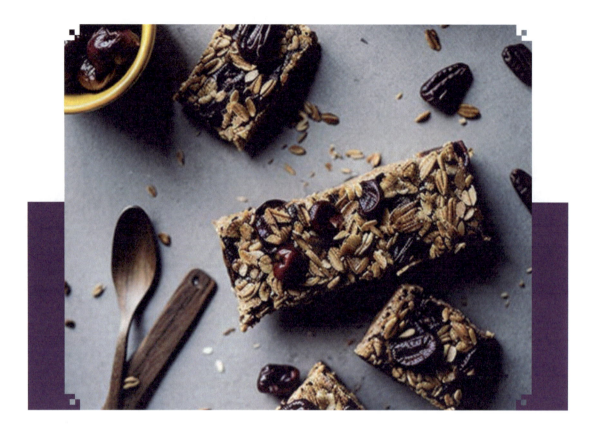

Cajun Spiced Pecans

Prep time: 5 minutes | Cook time: 30 minutes | Serves 4

- ½ pound pecan halves
- ½ tablespoon chilli powder
- ¼ teaspoon cayenne pepper
- ¼ teaspoon garlic powder
- 1 teaspoon dried thyme
- 1 tablespoon olive oil
- 1 teaspoon dried oregano

1. Place all the ingredients in the Instant Pot.
2. Select "Manual cook" and cook for 20 minutes at low pressure.
3. Release the pressure naturally and serve.

Cherry Pecan Granola Bars

Prep time: 10 minutes | Cook time: 15 minutes | Makes 12 bars

- 2 cups rolled oats
- ½ cup dates, pitted and coarsely chopped
- 1 cup fruit-sweetened dried cherries
- ¼ teaspoon ground allspice
- pinch salt, or to taste

1. Preheat the oven to 325°F.
2. Spread the oats on a 13 × 18-inch baking sheet and bake for 10 minutes, or until they start to brown.
3. Press the mixture into a nonstick 8 × 8-inch baking pan and bake for 20 minutes, or until the top is lightly golden.
4. Let cool before slicing into bars.

From Garden to Table

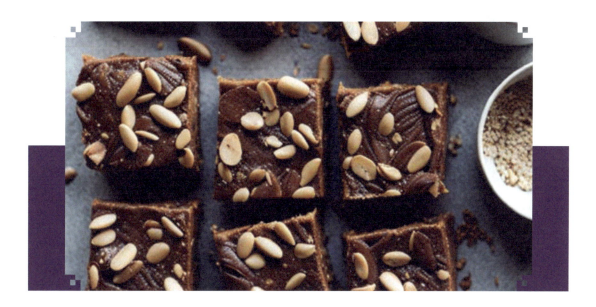

Mixed Berry Cobbler

Prep time: 10 minutes | Cook time: 15 minutes | Serves 9

- 1 teaspoon canola or vegetable oil (for greasing)
- 1 (12-ounce) bag frozen mixed berries
- ⅔ cup granulated sugar
- 1 cup whole wheat or all-purpose flour
- 2 teaspoons baking powder
- 1 cup plant-based milk

1. Preheat the oven to 375 degrees, and lightly grease an 8 × 8-inch baking pan.
2. In a medium bowl, thoroughly mix the frozen berries and sugar with a spoon. Set aside.
3. In a separate large bowl, thoroughly mix the flour, baking powder, milk, and butter with a spoon.
4. Spread the batter in the prepared pan.
5. Add the berry and sugar mixture on top of the batter.
6. Bake for 50 minutes or until golden.

Peanut Butter Snack Squares

Prep time: 20 minutes | Cook time: 35 minutes | Serves 8

- ½ cup coconut sugar
- 1 cup creamy peanut butter
- 1 teaspoon vanilla extract
- ¾ cup whole wheat flour
- ¼ cup garbanzo flour
- 1 teaspoon baking soda
- ½ teaspoon baking powder

1. Preheat the oven to 350°F. Lightly grease an 8-inch square baking dish.
2. Fold in the peanuts and dates and make sure everything is well incorporated.
3. You can use your hands to press the dough lightly into the prepared dish. Bake for 15 to 20 minutes or until lightly golden brown.
4. Place on a wire rack to cool. Cut into sixteen squares and store in the refrigerator.

Chapter 6

Burgers, Patties and Savory Cakes

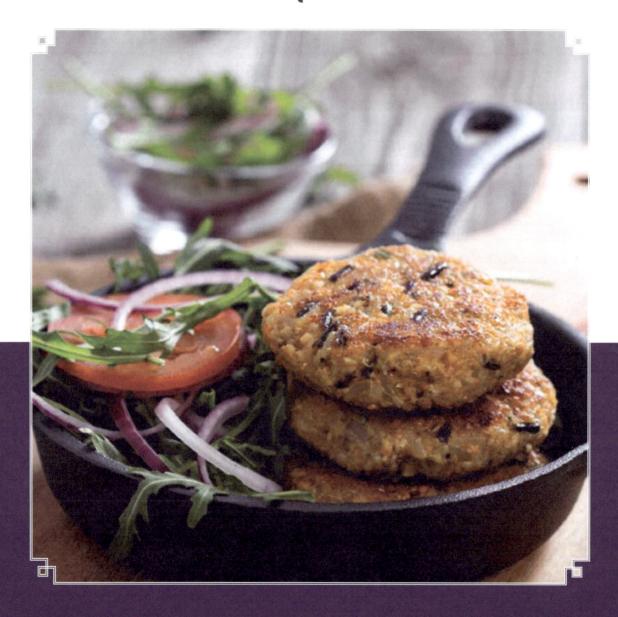

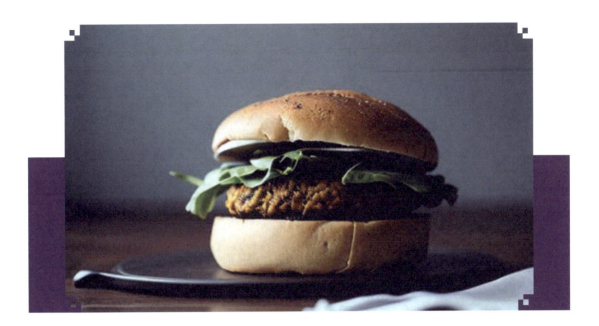

Black Beans Burger

Prep time: 15 minutes | **Cook time:** 5 minutes | Serves 5

- 1 cup black beans, cooked
- 2 tbsp bread crumbs
- 1 tsp salt
- ¼ cup sweet corn, cooked
- 1 tsp turmeric
- 1 tbsp fresh parsley, chopped
- ½ yellow sweet pepper, chopped
- ½ cup of water

1. Mash the black beans until you get purée and combine together with salt, sweet corn, turmeric, parsley, and sweet pepper.
2. Mix it up carefully with the help of a spoon.
3. Add bread crumbs and stir again.
4. Remove the foil from the burgers and transfer on the plate. Garnish burgers with lettuce leaves if desired.

Chickpea Burgers

Prep time: 5 minutes | **Cook time:** 15 minutes | Serves 2

- 1 (19-ounce) can chickpeas, drained
- ½ cup vegan bread crumbs
- ⅛ cup aquafaba (the liquid from a can of chickpeas)
- 2 tablespoons chickpea flour
- 1 tablespoon low-sodium soy sauce (or tamari, which is a gluten-free option)
- ⅛ teaspoon freshly ground black pepper

1. In a food processor, combine all the ingredients and pulse until roughly blended.
2. Using your hands, form the mixture into 2 patties.
3. In a nonstick pan over medium heat, cook the patties on each side for 5 minutes, or until lightly browned.
4. Serve on a whole-grain bun or lettuce wrap with your favorite condiments.

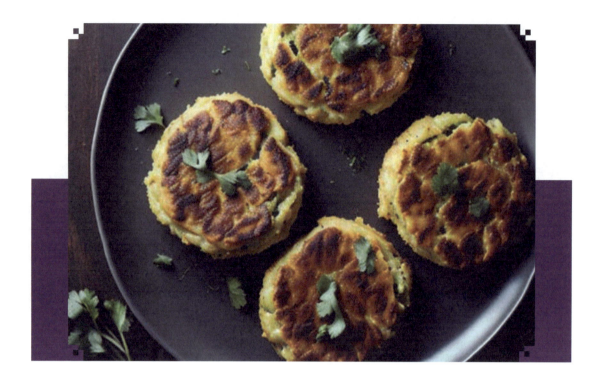

Dundee Cake

Prep time: 16 minutes | Cook time: 30 minutes | Serves 8

- cooking spray
- 4 tablespoons coconut oil
- 1/2 cup sugar
- 1 cup dried currants
- 1/3 cup slivered almonds
- 1 tablespoon grated orange peel
- 1 tablespoon grated lemon peel
- 1 cup self-rising flour

1. Spray the air fryer baking pan with nonstick cooking spray.
2. Preheat the air fryer to 330°F.
3. In a large bowl, mix together the egg replacer and water.
4. Stir in the coconut oil and sugar and beat until smooth.

Country Potato Patties

Prep time: 15 minutes (need cooked potatoes) | Cook time: 10 minutes | Serves 4

- 3 large potatoes, peeled or unpeeled, boiled until soft
- 2 tablespoons finely chopped onion
- 2 tablespoons finely chopped celery
- 2 tablespoons finely chopped green bell pepper
- 2 tablespoons whole-wheat flour
- 1 tablespoon minced fresh parsley

1. Shred the potatoes in a food processor or with a grater. Combine with the remaining ingredients and shape into four patties.
2. Cook on a nonstick griddle until browned on both sides, about 10 minutes.

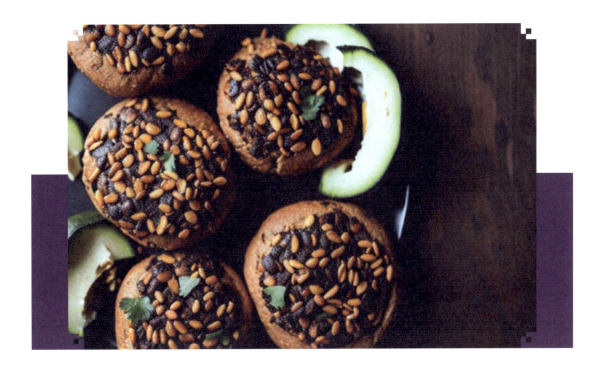

Cornmeal Cake

Prep time: 5 minutes | Cook time: 45 to 50 minutes | Serves 4 to 7

- 4 1/4 cups water
- 1/2 teaspoon salt (optional)
- 1 1/2 cups coarse cornmeal or polenta

1. Heat 2 cups of the water and the salt in a large saucepan until boiling furiously. Add the cornmeal to the remaining 2 1/2 cups cold water. Mix and add to the boiling water, stirring constantly.
2. Variations: Add 1/3 cup uncooked millet to the mixture after it thickens, just before covering and cooking for 30 to 40 minutes.
3. Add 1 cup frozen corn kernels about 10 minutes before the end of the final cooking time.

The Best Veggie Burgers

Prep time: 15 minutes | Cook time: 30 minutes | Serves 6

- 1 yellow onion, coarsely chopped
- 3 garlic cloves, coarsely chopped
- 1 sweet potato, skin on, cubed
- ½ cup walnuts
- 1 cup precooked brown rice
- 2 cups precooked green lentils or brown lentils
- ¼ cup ground flaxseed
- ¾ to 1 cup coarse cornmeal

1. Preheat the oven to 450°F. Line a baking sheet with parchment paper.
2. In a food processor, combine the onion, garlic, sweet potato, and walnuts. Process for 1 to 2 minutes, or until the ingredients are combined and have the consistency of rice.

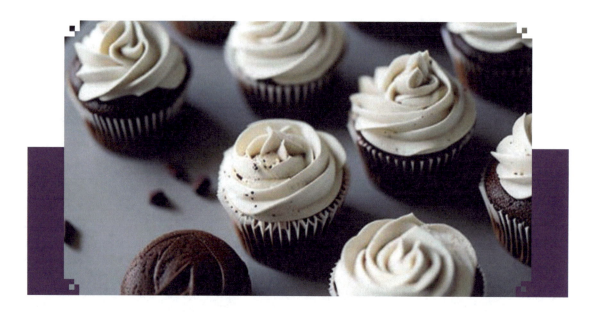

Almond Berry Cake

Prep time: 10 minutes | Cook time: 35 minutes | Serves 6

- 1 cup nondairy milk
- 1 tsp apple cider vinegar
- 1 tsp almond extract
- 1½ cups gluten-free baking mix
- ½ cup vegan sugar
- 1 tbsp ground flaxseed
- ½ tsp baking powder
- ½ tsp baking soda

1. Oil a pan that fits into your Instant Pot or cover in parchment paper to keep oil-free. In a large measuring cup, combine the nondairy milk, vinegar and almond extract.
2. In a small mixing bowl, combine the baking mix, sugar, ground flaxseed, baking powder, baking soda and salt.
3. To make handles out of aluminum foil: Pull the handles up and carefully lift the pan or container into your Instant Pot.

Depression Era Cupcakes

Prep time: 10 minutes | Cook time: 15 minutes | Makes 12 cupcakes

- 1½ cups whole wheat or all-purpose flour
- ¾–1 cup granulated sugar (depending on your sweet tooth)
- 3 tablespoons cocoa powder
- 1 teaspoon baking soda
- ½ teaspoon salt
- 1 teaspoon vanilla extract
- 1 teaspoon white or apple cider vinegar
- 5 tablespoons canola or vegetable oil
- 1 cup water

1. Preheat the oven to 350 degrees. Line a cupcake tin with paper baking cups.
2. In the bowl of an electric mixer (or in a large bowl, by hand), mix together all the ingredients until smooth.
3. Bake for 15 to 20 minutes. Test a cupcake by sticking a toothpick in the middle. If the toothpick comes out dry, the cupcakes are done.

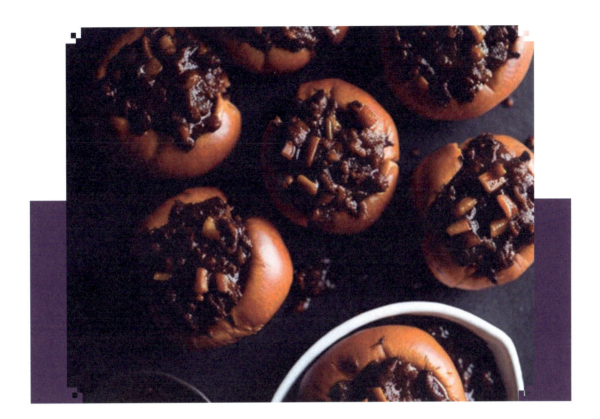

Sloppy Cajun Burgers

Prep time: 30 minutes | Cook time: 5 minutes| Serves 4

- 1 cup black beans
- 1 7-oz pack textured soy mince
- 1 cup tomato cubes
- ¼ cup salt-free cajun spices
- 4 whole wheat buns
- dill pickle slices
- whole wheat buns (gluten)

1. Put a non-stick deep frying pan over medium high heat and add the soy mince, and the tomato cubes.
2. Let it cook for about 3 minutes, stirring occasionally with a spatula, until everything is cooked.

Seitan Sloppy Joes

Prep time: 20 minutes | Cook time: 35 minutes | Serves 6

- 2 cups seitan, crumbled (slow cooker log for thin slices and crumbles)
- 8 ounces tomato sauce
- ⅓ cup organic ketchup
- 1 tablespoon vegan worcestershire sauce
- 2 tablespoons red wine vinegar
- 2 tablespoons coconut sugar
- 6 toasted whole wheat buns

1. Add all of the ingredients except the buns to a large skillet. Bring to a boil, then turn the heat down to medium.
2. Cook for 15 minutes. Serve on the toasted buns.

Chapter 7

Rice, Grains, Potatoes Perfected

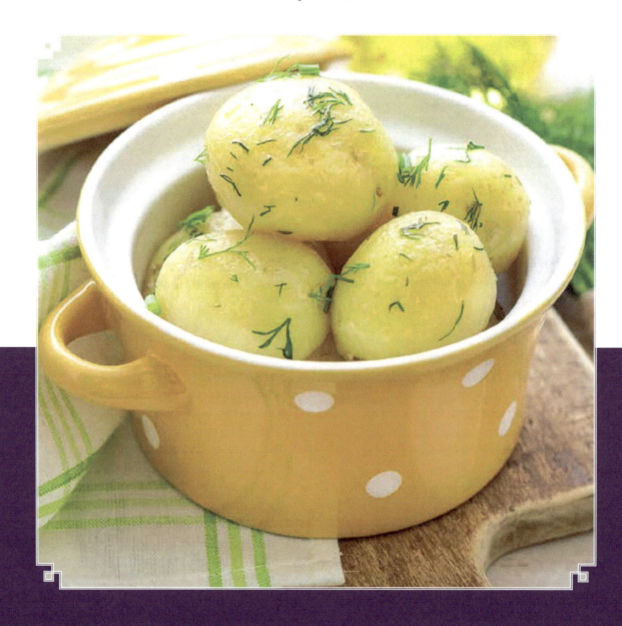

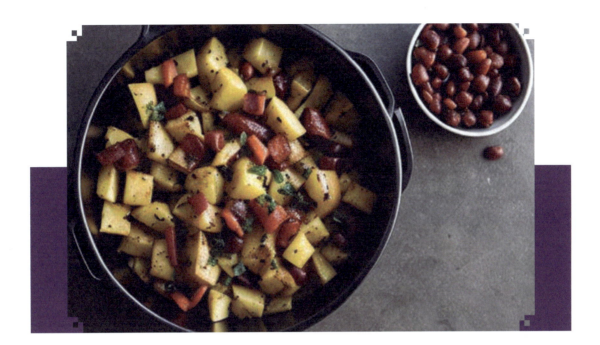

Broccoli-Rice Casserole

Prep time: 15 minutes | Cook time: 20 minutes | Serves 8

- oil for misting or cooking spray
- 1 (16-ounce) package soft silken tofu
- 1/2 cup Cheddar-style shreds
- 1 teaspoon salt
- 2 tablespoons almond milk
- 1 (12-ounce) package chopped broccoli, thawed
- 1 cup cooked rice

1. Spray the air fryer baking pan with oil or nonstick spray.
2. In a large bowl, beat together the tofu, cheese shreds, salt, and milk with an electric mixer until they combine.
3. Stir in the broccoli and rice.
4. Spoon the casserole mixture into the prepared baking pan.
5. Cook at 360°F for 20 minutes.

Breakfast Potatoes

Prep time: 10 minutes | Cook time: 35 minutes | Serves 5

- 6 medium potatoes, peeled and ½-inch cubed
- 1 medium white onion, peeled and ½-inch cubed
- 1 medium green bell pepper, ½-inch cubed
- 3/4 cup vegetable broth

1. Switch on the instant pot, add 3 tablespoons coconut oil in the inner pot, press the sauté/simmer button, then adjust cooking time to 5 minutes and let preheat.
2. Then add potatoes and cook for 3 minutes or until sauté.
3. Return vegetables into the pan, stir well and cook for 1 minute or until thoroughly heated.
4. Serve immediately.

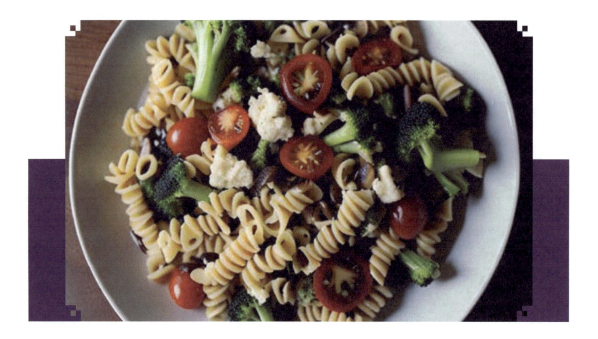

Rice and Noodle Pilaf

Prep time: 5 minutes | **Cook time:** 35 to 45 minutes | **Serves 6 to 8**

- 1 cup whole-wheat noodles
- 2 cups long-grain brown rice
- 6½ cups vegetable broth or water
- 1 teaspoon ground cumin
- ½ teaspoon dried oregano

1. Break the noodles up into very small pieces, about 1/8 inch long. (Put them in a towel or bag and crush with a rolling pin.)
2. Place them in a saucepan along with the rice. Heat over medium heat, stirring constantly, until they begin to smell toasted, 3 to 4 minutes. Add the liquid and the seasonings. Mix well.
3. Bring to a boil, cover, reduce the heat to medium-low, and cook until all water is absorbed, 30 to 40 minutes.

Garden Pasta Salad

Prep time: 30 minutes | **Cook time:** 2 hours | **Serves 8 to 10**

- 4 quarts water
- 1 cup chopped broccoli
- 1 cup chopped cauliflower
- ¾ cup cherry tomatoes, cut in half
- ¾ to 1 cup oil-free Italian dressing
- freshly ground black pepper to taste

1. Bring the water to a boil and add the pasta. Return to boiling and cook, uncovered, for 6 minutes. Drain. Rinse under cool water and set aside.
2. Place the broccoli, cauliflower, and snow peas in a steamer basket. Steam over boiling water for 4 to 5 minutes, until tender-crisp.
3. Combine all of the ingredients in a large bowl. Toss to mix well. Refrigerate for at least 2 hours before serving.

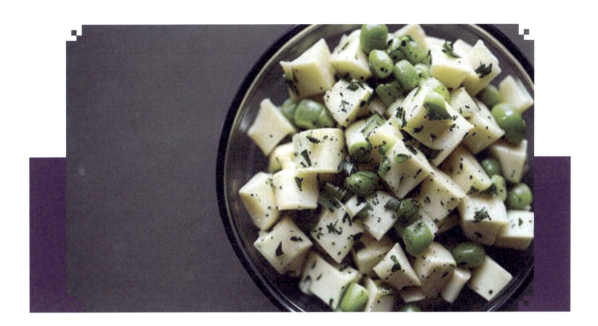

Mushroom Risotto

Prep time: 10 minutes | Cook time: 55 minutes | Serves 4

- 1 yellow onion, chopped
- 3 garlic cloves, minced
- ½ celery stalk, minced
- 1 tablespoon water, plus more as needed
- 9 ounces baby portabella mushrooms, coarsely chopped

1. In an 8-quart pot over high heat, combine the onion, garlic, and celery. Add the baby portabella and shiitake mushrooms and sauté for 3 to 4 minutes, stirring, until the liquid from the mushrooms evaporates.
2. Add the remaining 1½ cups of vegetable broth. Cook, stirring continuously but lightly, for 5 to 10 minutes more, or until the liquid has been mostly absorbed.
3. Stir in the red kidney beans. Serve warm, topped with scallions.

Potato Salad

Prep time: 10 minutes | Cook time: 15 minutes | Serves 4

- 6 medium potatoes, cubed and boiled
- ¾ cup Mighty Mayo
- 2 celery stalks, diced
- 2 or 3 scallions, chopped
- 2 dill pickles, chopped
- pink himalayan salt
- ground paprika (optional)

1. Cook the potatoes in boiling water for 15 minutes, or until tender but still a little firm. Drain and rinse the potatoes in cool water.
2. In a bowl, combine the potatoes, mayo, celery, scallions, pickles, and and salt to taste. Mix until thoroughly coated. Sprinkle with paprika (if using). Enjoy immediately or store in a reusable container in the refrigerator for up to 5 days.

From Garden to Table

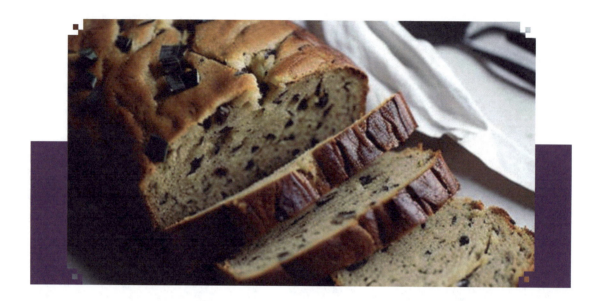

White Bean Veggie Wrap

Prep time: 5 minutes | Cook time: 10 minutes | Serves 4

- 1 red onion, diced
- 1 red bell pepper, diced
- 1 medium zucchini, diced
- 1 medium yellow squash, diced
- Sea salt and black pepper to taste
- 4 12-inch whole-grain flatbreads
- 1 cup White Bean Spread or hummus
- ½ cup chopped fresh basil

1. Heat a large skillet over high heat. Add the onion, red bell pepper, zucchini, and yellow squash, and stir-fry until the onion is translucent and the vegetables start to brown, about 5 to 6 minutes.
2. Top with sautéed vegetables and some of the chopped basil.
3. Fold in the top half of one flatbread over the vegetable mixture, fold in the sides, and roll the wrap up like a cigar.
4. Repeat with the remaining flatbreads.

Zucchini Bread

Prep time: 25 minutes | Cook time: 1¼ hours | Serves One 8 × 4-inch loaf

- ¼ cup mashed banana (about 1 medium banana)
- 1 tablespoon fresh lemon juice
- 1 teaspoon vanilla extract
- 2 cups whole-wheat pastry flour
- ½ teaspoon baking soda
- 2 teaspoons baking powder
- 1 teaspoon grated lemon zest
- 2 teaspoons ground cinnamon
- ½ cup raisins

1. Preheat the oven to 350°F.
2. In a large bowl, combine the banana, zucchini, juices, and vanilla. Pour the wet ingredients into the dry and mix thoroughly.
3. Pour into a nonstick 8 × 4-inch loaf until a toothpick inserted in the center comes out clean. Cool completely on a rack.

Chapter 8

Soups, Stews, and Chilis

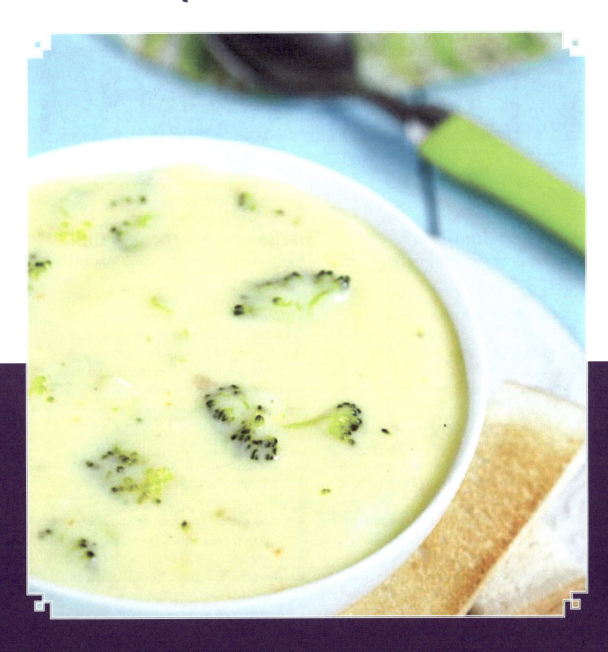

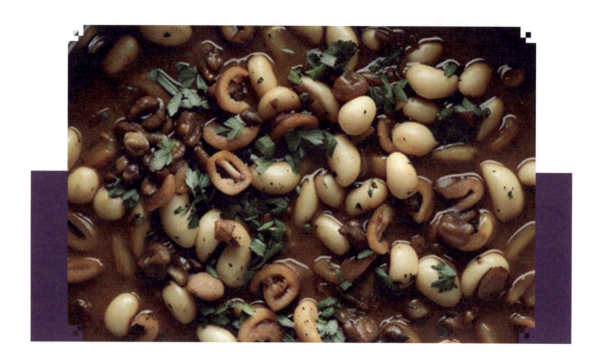

Split Pea Soup

Prep time: 10 minutes| Cook time: 20 minutes| Serves 4

- 2 cups yellow split peas, uncooked
- 1 medium white onion, peeled and diced
- 2 stalks celery, sliced
- 3 medium carrots, sliced
- 1 ½ teaspoon minced garlic

1. Switch on the instant pot, grease the inner pot with 1 tablespoon olive oil, press the sauté/simmer button, then adjust cooking time to 5 minutes and let preheat.
2. Add onion, cook for 1 minute, then add carrot, garlic, and celery and cook for 2 minutes or until sauté.
3. Then carefully open the instant pot, stir the soup, garnish with parsley and serve.

Bean and Mushroom Chili

Prep time: 10 minutes | Cook time: 15 minutes | Serves 6

- 1 large onion, peeled and chopped
- 1 pound button mushrooms, chopped
- 6 cloves garlic, peeled and minced
- 1 tablespoon ground cumin
- 1 tablespoon ancho chile powder
- 4 teaspoons ground fennel
- salt to taste

1. Place the onion and mushrooms in a large saucepan and sauté over medium heat for 10 minutes.
2. Add water 1 to 2 tablespoons at a time to keep the vegetables from sticking to the pan.
3. Add the tomatoes, beans, and 2 cups minutes.
4. Season with salt.

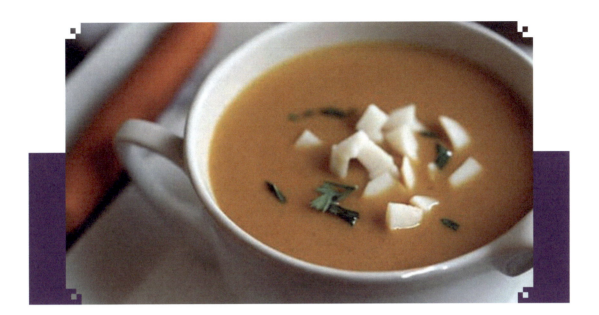

Roasted Veggie Soup

Prep time: 10 minutes | Cook time: 7 minutes | Serves 1

- 8 small red potatoes, halved
- 2 cups chopped cauliflower
- 1 cup chopped broccoli
- 1 tbsp olive oil
- 1 tsp kosher salt
- 1 tsp freshly ground black pepper
- 3 cups low-Sodium: vegetable broth

1. Set the air fryer temp to 400°F.
2. Place the potatoes in a microwave-safe bowl and cover with water. Microwave the potatoes until tender, about 4 to 5 minutes.
3. Drain the water and place the potatoes in a large bowl. Add the cauliflower, broccoli, olive oil, salt, and pepper. Toss well to coat.
4. Transfer the soup to bowls and serve immediately with the whole grain crackers.

Sweet Squash Soup

Prep time: 30 minutes | Cook time: 45 minutes | Serves 8 to 10

- 1 large butternut or buttercup squash
- 1 1/2 cups sliced onion
- 1 1/2 cups peeled and chopped apple
- 1 cup chopped carrot
- 2 to 3 teaspoons minced fresh ginger
- 5 cups water

1. Put the whole squash in a microwave oven and cook on high power for 8 minutes. Peel the squash and cut into cubes. (If you don't have a microwave oven, this step may be omitted. This brief cooking time simply makes the squash easier to peel and cut up.)
2. Place all of the ingredients in a large soup pot and simmer over medium-low heat for 45 minutes. Place the soup in a blender or food processor, in batches, and blend until smooth and creamy.

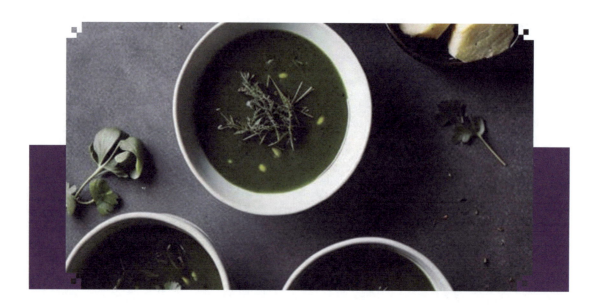

Kale White Bean Soup

Prep time: 20 minutes | Cook time: 10 hours 20 minutes | Serves 6

- 1 pound navy beans
- 1 tablespoon coconut oil
- ½ cup coarsely chopped onions
- 1 clove garlic, minced
- ¼ cup nutritional yeast
- 1 red bell pepper, diced
- 4 roma tomatoes, chopped
- 1 pound kale, de-stemmed and coarsely chopped

1. Place the beans in a large stockpot and cover with water by about 3 inches. If you want to do the quick method for preparing the beans—instead of soaking overnight—then cover beans with water by 2 inches in the stockpot.
2. Stir in kale and 2 cups water and simmer, uncovered, until kale is tender, about 12 to 15 minutes.

Watercress-Potato Soup

Prep time: 5 minutes | Cook time: 45 minutes | Serves 4-6

- 2 large leeks, diced
- 3 cloves garlic, minced
- 1 teaspoon minced fresh thyme
- 4 large potatoes, peeled and diced
- 2 bunches watercress, chopped
- Sea salt and pepper to taste

1. Sauté the leeks in a large saucepan over medium heat until softened, about 8 minutes.
2. Add water 1 to 2 tablespoons at a time to keep them from sticking.
3. Add the garlic and thyme, and cook for 2 minutes.
4. Add the potatoes and vegetable stock, and bring to a boil.
5. Purée the soup in batches in a blender and return to a pan over low heat.
6. Season with salt and pepper and cook for another 5 minutes.

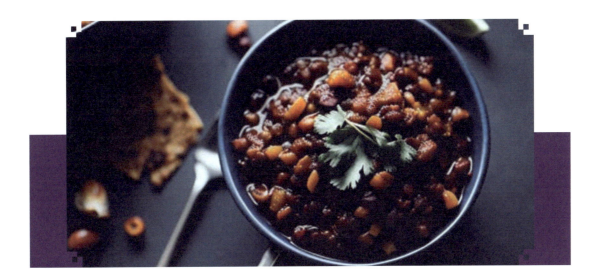

Pumpkin and Anasazi Bean Stew

Prep time: 10 minutes | **Cook time:** 15 minutes | Serves 6 to 8

- 1 large yellow onion, peeled and diced
- 2 large carrots, peeled and diced
- 2 celery stalks, diced
- 2 cloves garlic, peeled and minced
- 2 tablespoons cumin seeds, toasted and ground
- 2 tablespoons tomato paste
- 6 green onions (white and green parts), thinly sliced

1. Place the onion, carrots, and celery in a large saucepan and sauté over medium heat for 10 minutes.
2. Add water 1 to 2 tablespoons at a time to keep the vegetables from sticking to the pan.
3. Add the garlic and cook for another minute.
4. Season with salt and pepper and serve garnished with the green onions.

Extra-Spicy Lentil Chili

Prep time: 15 minutes | **Cook time:** 30 to 35 minutes | Serves 6 to 8

- 1 pound lentils
- 2 quarts vegetable broth or water
- 2 cups diced onion
- 1 cup crushed tomatoes
- $\frac{1}{4}$ cup tomato paste
- 2 tablespoons chopped garlic
- 2 tablespoons balsamic vinegar
- 2 tablespoons fresh lime juice
- 1 tablespoon ground cumin
- 2 tablespoons chili powder
- 1 teaspoon cayenne (use less if you don't like your chili spicy)

1. Combine all of the ingredients in a large soup pot. Bring to a boil over high heat.
2. Reduce the heat, cover, and simmer over medium-low heat until the lentils are tender, 30 to 35 minutes, adding more water or broth if needed for proper chili consistency.

Chapter 9

Meal Helpers, Veggie Sides, Dips

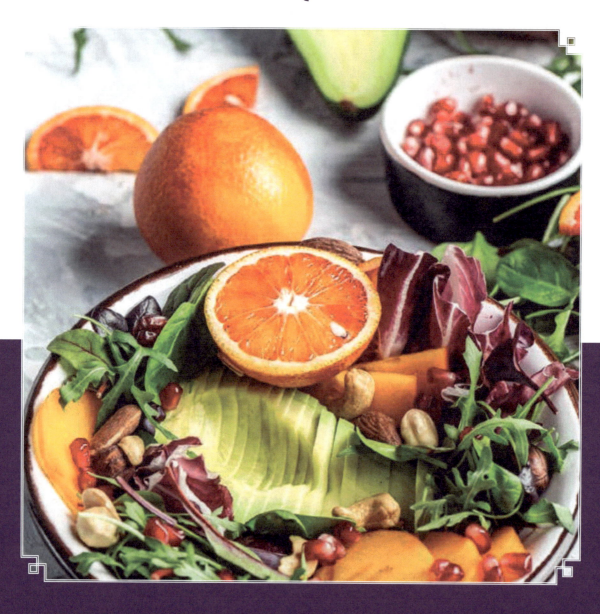

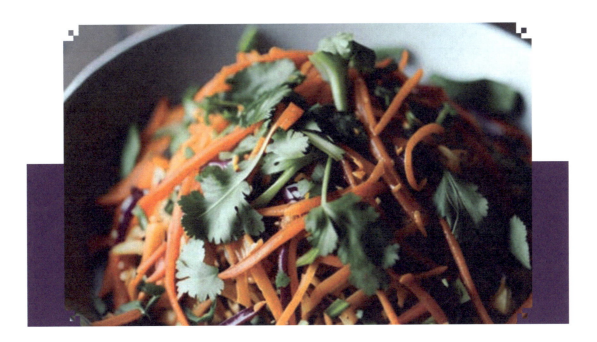

Rosemary and Thyme Brussels Sprouts

Prep time: 5 minutes | **Cook time:** 10 minutes | Serves 4

- 1 pound Brussels sprouts
- 1 teaspoon whole rosemary leaves
- 1 teaspoon dried thyme leaves
- 1 tablespoon walnut oil
- 1 tablespoon coarsely chopped garlic
- 1/4 teaspoon sea salt
- 1 cup water
- 1 teaspoon balsamic vinegar (optional)

1. Wash the brussels sprouts and remove the stems with a knife; the loose outer leaves should come off easily. Cut each in half. Set aside.
2. Cover and bring to pressure. Cook at high pressure for 1 minute. Use a quick release.
3. Remove the lid, stir in the balsamic vinegar, and serve immediately.

Thai Cabbage Salad

Prep time: 30 minutes | **Cook time:** 35 minutes | Serves 6 to 8

- 2 cloves garlic
- 2 to 4 small red chili peppers
- 6 1/2 tablespoons fresh lime juice
- 4 tablespoons soy sauce
- 1/2 head green cabbage, shredded
- 1/2 head red cabbage, shredded
- 2 to 3 large carrots, scrubbed and grated
- 1 cup lettuce leaves

1. Grind the garlic and chilies in a small food processor or with a mortar and pestle. Pour the lime juice and soy sauce into a small jar. Add the chili paste and shake well to mix. Set aside.
2. Place the shredded cabbage and carrot in a large bowl. Mix well. Pour the dressing over the vegetables and toss to mix. Serve on a bed of lettuce.

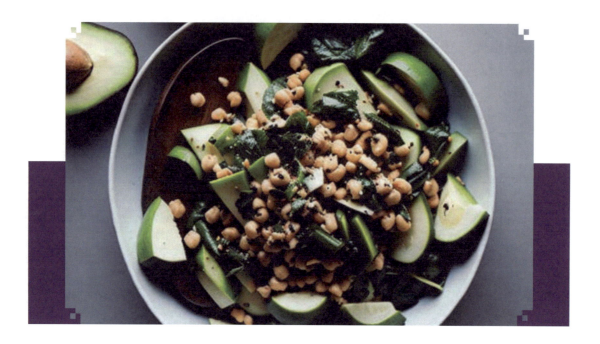

Italian Farro Salad

Prep time: 15 minutes | Cook time: 40 minutes | Serves 6

- 1 cup farro, rinsed and drained
- 3 cups water
- 4 roma tomatoes, deseeded and diced
- 1 clove garlic, minced
- sea salt, to taste
- freshly ground black pepper, to taste

1. Add the farro and 3 cups water to the inner pot. Lock the lid and ensure the steam release valve is set to the sealing position. Select Pressure Cook (High), and set the cook time for 17 minutes.
2. To prepare the salad, add the diced to a salad bowl. Add the cooked and cooled farro, and toss to combine.
3. In a small bowl, whisk together the lettuce, drizzled with a bit more oil and vinegar.

Sesame Celery Bowl

Prep time: 10 minutes | Cook time: 15 minutes | Serves 2

- 2 cups fresh spinach
- 1 can (15 ounces) chickpeas, rinsed and drained
- 2 ribs celery, very thinly sliced
- 2 carrots, shredded
- ½ cucumber, thinly sliced
- 2 scallions, thinly sliced
- 1 ripe avocado, diced
- 4 tablespoons sliced almonds
- 2 tablespoons spicy dressing

1. Place 1 cup of spinach each in 2 bowls. To each bowl, add half of the chickpeas, celery, carrots, cucumber, scallions, and avocado.
2. Sprinkle the sliced almonds on top. Drizzle 1 tablespoon of dressing over each bowl and serve.

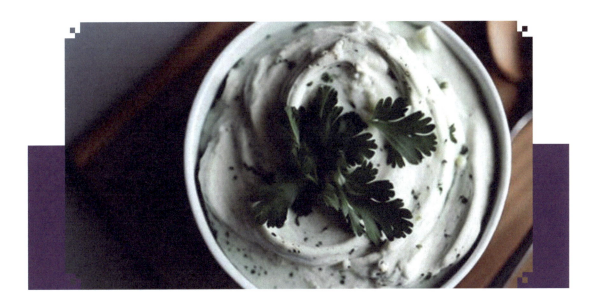

Tempeh Chickpea Stuffed Mini Peppers

Prep time: 20 minutes | **Cook time:** 35 minutes | Serves 6

- ¾ cup tempeh, chopped
- ½ cup dairy-free mayonnaise
- ¼ cup cider vinegar
- 1 teaspoon ground mustard
- 3 scallions, thinly sliced
- 1 teaspoon salt
- ¼ teaspoon cayenne pepper

1. Cut off the stem end of the peppers. Slice lengthwise. Remove any seeds that are inside. Set aside.
2. Place all the remaining ingredients in a food processor. Pulse four or five times. The chickpeas should be chunky. Remove the blade and stir to make sure the mixture is blended well.
3. Stuff each pepper half full with about 2 tablespoons of the chickpea mixture. Set on a plate to serve.

Cucumber Dip

Prep time: 10 minutes | **Cook time:** 15 minutes | Makes 1½ cups

- 1 cucumber
- 1 cup plain soy yogurt
- 3 to 4 cloves garlic, crushed
- ¼ teaspoon white pepper, or to taste

1. Peel the cucumber and cut it in half lengthwise. Scoop out and discard the seeds; coarsely chop the cucumber. Place it in a food processor and chop very fine. (This may also be done with a hand grater.)
2. Remove from the food processor and place in a very fine strainer. Press out as much water as possible. Return to the food processor (or place in a blender). Add the remaining ingredients and process until fairly smooth. Add more garlic and/or white pepper to taste. Refrigerate for several hours before using, for best flavor.

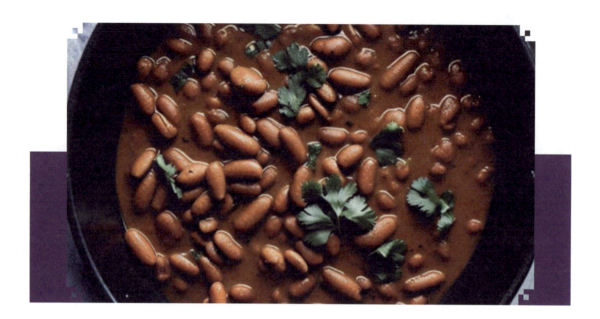

Corn Salad

Prep time: 18 minutes | Cook time: 12 minutes | Serves 6

- 1 tablespoon light olive oil
- 1/2 teaspoon garlic powder
- 1/2 teaspoon cumin
- 2 small ears corn
- 1 cup cooked black beans
- 1/2 cup slivered poblano peppers
- 1/2 medium red or white onion
- 1 small avocado
- 3 tablespoons lime juice
- 1/4 teaspoon salt

1. In a small bowl, mix the olive oil, garlic powder, and cumin.
2. Remove the husks and silk from the ears of corn.
3. Dice the avocado into 1/4-inch cubes.
4. Toss the corn, beans, peppers, onion, and avocado together with the lime juice and salt.

Smashed Beans

Prep time: 10 minutes, plus overnight soaking | Cook time: 3 to 4 hours (or all day in a slow cooker) | Makes about 6 cups

- 2 cups pinto beans
- 8 cups water
- 1/2 teaspoon onion powder
- 1/2 teaspoon garlic powder
- 1/2 to 1 cup mild or spicy salsa

1. Place the beans in a large pot with the water. Bring to a boil, cover, reduce the heat, and cook until tender, 3 to 4 hours. (To reduce the cooking time, soak the beans overnight in the water. Then proceed as directed, reducing cooking time by 1/2 hour.) Drain, reserving the cooking liquid.
2. Mash the beans, using a hand masher, electric beater, or food processor. smashed consistency. Heat through to blend the flavors.

From Garden to Table

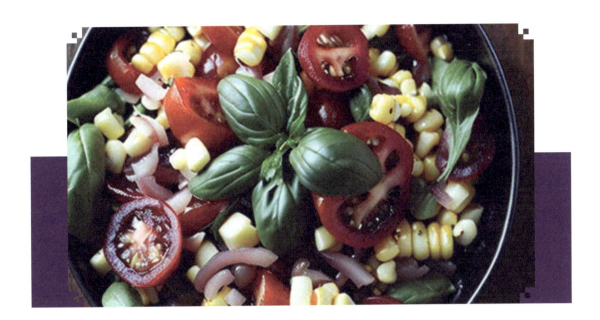

Golden Spicy Cauliflower

Prep time: 15 minutes | Cook time: 20 minutes | Serves 4 to 6

- 1 medium cauliflower, cut into florets
- 2 cloves garlic, pressed
- 2 to 3 tablespoons grated fresh ginger
- 1 cup water
- 2 medium tomatoes, seeded and chopped
- 1 bunch scallions, chopped

1. Place the cauliflower, garlic, and ginger in a saucepan with 1/2 cup of the water. Cook, stirring occasionally, for about 10 minutes.
2. Add the remaining water and the rest of the ingredients. Bring to a boil, reduce the heat, and simmer, covered, until the cauliflower is tender, about 10 minutes longer.
3. Stir occasionally during cooking to prevent the cauliflower from sticking to the bottom of the pan.

Tomato, Corn and Bean Salad

Prep time: 10 minutes | Cook time: 15 minutes | Serves 4

- 6 ears corn
- 3 large tomatoes, diced
- 2 cups cooked navy beans, or one 15-ounce can, drained and rinsed
- 1 cup finely chopped basil
- 2 tablespoons balsamic vinegar
- salt and freshly ground black pepper to taste

1. Bring a large pot of water to a boil.
2. Add the corn and cook for 7 to 10 minutes.
3. Drain the water from the pot and rinse the corn under cold water to cool, then cut the kernels from the cob.
4. In a large bowl, toss together the corn, tomatoes, beans, onion, basil, balsamic vinegar, and salt and pepper.
5. Chill for 1 hour before serving.

Chapter 10

Divine Desserts and Drinks

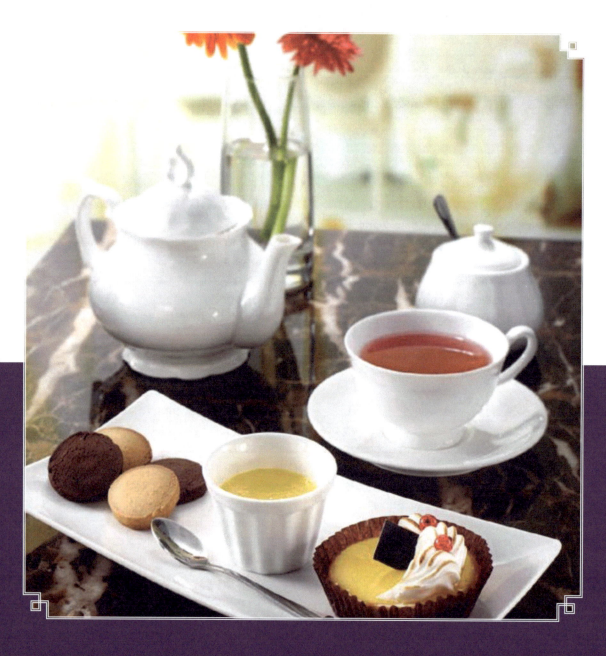

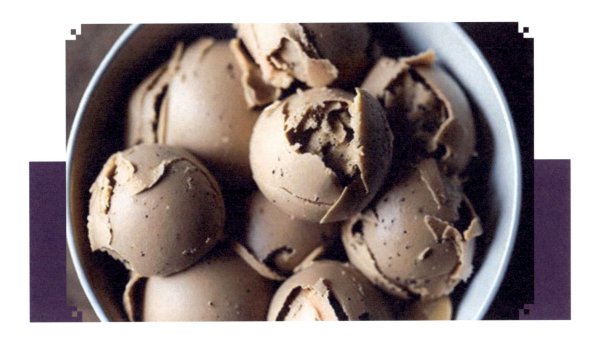

Mini Berry Tarts

Prep time: 5 minutes| Cook time: 1 minute | Serves 6

- 2 cups blueberries, sliced strawberries, and raspberries
- 1/3 cup lemon juice
- 1/8 tsp salt
- ½ cup beet sugar
- 2 tbsp cornstarch
- 1 ¼ cups whipped coconut cream
- 15 medium phyllo shells, thawed

1. Turn on, open the instant pot, and select Sauté mode.
2. Pour in the berries, lemon juice, salt, beet sugar, combine the cornstarch with the water and add to the pot.
3. After, remove the tarts, top with the whipped coconut cream, and then garnish with a combination of fresh berries.

Banana Ice Cream

Prep time: 10 minutes | Cook time: 15 minutes | Serves 4

- 4 ripe bananas, cut into 2-inch pieces
- ¼ cup almond butter
- 1 tablespoon pure vanilla extract
- pinch of ground cinnamon
- pinch of sea salt

1. Freeze the banana pieces for at least 4 hours.
2. In a high-powered blender, combine the bananas, almond butter, vanilla, cinnamon, and salt. Blend, stopping to push the bananas down and scrape down the sides. Or the mixture can be frozen until firm enough to scoop.
3. Serve in a bowl with the crackle sauce, if using. Store leftovers in an airtight container in the freezer for up to 2 weeks.

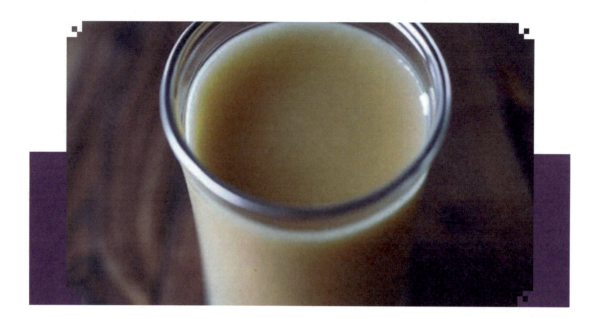

Salted Caramel Bites

Prep time: 10 minutes | Cook time: 15 minutes | Makes 18 bites

- 1 cup raw cashews
- 1 cup soft and sticky medjool dates, pitted
- ½ cup tahini
- 1 teaspoon pure vanilla extract
- ¼ teaspoon sea salt

1. In the bowl of a food processor fitted with the chopping blade, pulse the cashews until finely chopped. Add the dates and process until a thick, sticky paste forms. Stop to scrape down the sides of the bowl as needed.
2. Scoop out a heaping teaspoon of the mixture and roll into a ball about 1½ inches in diameter. Repeat to form approximately 18 balls. Freeze on a baking sheet until firm, then transfer to an airtight container and store at room temperature for up to 5 days.

Lemon Curd

Prep time: 10 minutes | Cook time: 10 minutes | Serves 2

- ½ cup lemon juice
- 1 cup of coconut milk
- 1 teaspoon lemon zest
- 1 tablespoon cornstarch
- ¾ cup brown sugar

1. Preheat instant pot on Saute mode.
2. Meanwhile, whisk together lemon juice and cornstarch.
3. Then pour coconut milk in the preheated instant pot.
4. Add lemon juice mixture, lemon zest, and vanilla extract. Whisk it gently to make the homogenous liquid.
5. Then add sugar and start to stir it constantly until the liquid is thick. The curd is cooked.
6. Strain it with the help of colander and transfer in the serving bowls.

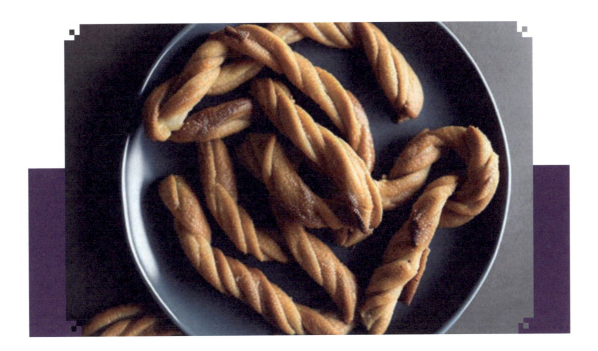

Oatberry Yogurt Muffins

Prep time: 10 minutes | **Cook time:** 15 minutes | Makes 12 muffins

- 2¼ cups oat flour
- 1 tablespoon baking powder
- ¾ teaspoon salt
- ½ cup dry sweetener
- ½ cup unsweetened applesauce
- ½ cup unsweetened plain soy yogurt
- 2 teaspoons pure vanilla extract

1. Preheat the oven to 350°F.
2. Line a 12-cup muffin pan with silicone liners or have ready a nonstick or silicone muffin pan (see recommendations).
3. Let the muffins cool completely, about 20 minutes, then carefully run a knife around the edges of each muffin to remove.

Cinnamon Twists

Prep time: 10 minutes | **Cook time:** 12 minutes | Serves 2

- 2 cups all-purpose flour, plus more
- ½ tsp kosher salt
- ½ cup canola oil
- 5 to 8 tbsp cold water
- ¼ cup granulated sugar
- 1½ tsp ground cinnamon

1. Set the air fryer temp to 330°F.
2. In a medium bowl, combine the flour and salt.
3. In a small bowl, combine the sugar and cinnamon.
4. Working in batches, place 10 twists in the fryer basket and cook until golden brown, about 5 to 6 minutes.
5. Transfer the cinnamon twists to a platter and allow to cool slightly before serving.

From Garden to Table

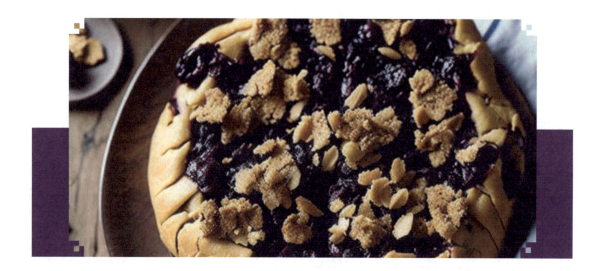

English Muffin Protein Triangles

Prep time: 20 minutes | Cook time: 1 hour 20 minutes | Serves 6

- 3 english muffins
- 1½ tablespoons lemon juice
- 1½ tablespoons nutritional yeast
- 1 teaspoon curry powder
- ½ teaspoon mustard powder
- ½ teaspoon salt
- pinch of ground black pepper
- ¼ cup black olives, sliced
- freshly cut parsley, for garnish (optional)

1. Break apart the English muffins at the center and toast. Place on a baking sheet and set aside.
2. Divide the mixture and spread on the six muffin halves. It will be thick. Slide the baking sheet under the broiler for about 2 minutes, until lightly golden.
3. Top with black olive slices and cut each muffin into quarters. Stack on a plate and garnish with freshly cut parsley, if desired.

Blueberry Crisp

Prep time: 10 minutes | Cook time: 17 minutes | Serves 4

- 2 cups fresh blueberries
- juice of ½ orange
- 1 tbsp maple syrup
- 2 tsp cornstarch
- 1 tbsp vegan butter
- ½ cup rolled oats
- ¼ cup almond flour
- ½ tsp ground cinnamon
- 2 tbsp coconut sugar or granulated sugar
- pinch of kosher salt

1. Set the air fryer temp to 370°F.
2. In a baking dish, combine the blueberries, orange juice, maple syrup, and cornstarch. Mix well.
3. Place the dish in the fryer basket and bake until the topping is crispy and the berries are thick and bubbly, about 15 to 17 minutes.
4. Remove the dish from the fryer basket and allow the crisp to cool for at least 10 minutes before serving.

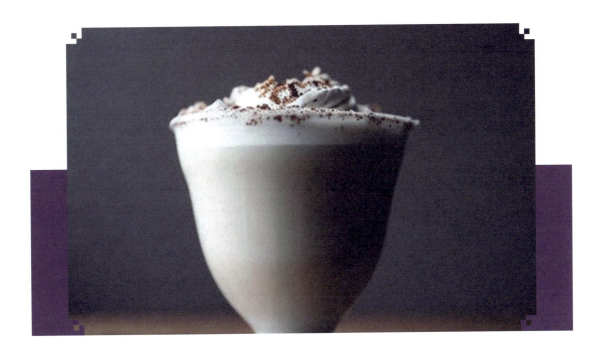

Summer Sangria

Prep time: 10 minutes | **Cook time:** 15 minutes | Serves 8

- 1 orange, very thinly sliced
- 1 green apple, cored and thinly sliced
- 1 ripe-firm white peach, thinly sliced
- 1 lemon, thinly sliced
- 1 lime, thinly sliced
- 1 pint raspberries
- fresh mint sprigs

1. In a 1-gallon pitcher or beverage container, combine the orange, apple, peach, lemon, lime, raspberries, and
2. Just before serving, add the sparkling water to the pitcher and stir. Fill 8 glasses with ice and pour sangria over the top. Transfer some of the fruit into the glasses, if desired, and garnish with mint sprigs.

Vanilla Steamer

Prep time: 10 minutes | **Cook time:** 15 minutes | Serves 1

- 1 cup unsweetened plain almond milk
- 2 teaspoons pure maple syrup
- ½ teaspoon pure vanilla extract
- pinch of ground cinnamon

1. In a small saucepan over medium heat, warm the almond milk for 5 minutes, or until very hot but not boiling.
2. Transfer the hot milk to a blender, then add the maple syrup and vanilla. Carefully blend on low speed for 10 seconds, then increase the speed to high and blend until frothy and well combined.
3. Pour into a heatproof mug, sprinkle with cinnamon, and enjoy immediately.

Appendix 1 Measurement Conversion Chart

Volume Equivalents (Dry)	
US STANDARD	METRIC (APPROXIMATE)
1/8 teaspoon	0.5 mL
1/4 teaspoon	1 mL
1/2 teaspoon	2 mL
3/4 teaspoon	4 mL
1 teaspoon	5 mL
1 tablespoon	15 mL
1/4 cup	59 mL
1/2 cup	118 mL
3/4 cup	177 mL
1 cup	235 mL
2 cups	475 mL
3 cups	700 mL
4 cups	1 L

Volume Equivalents (Liquid)		
US STANDARD	US STANDARD (OUNCES)	METRIC (APPROXIMATE)
2 tablespoons	1 fl.oz.	30 mL
1/4 cup	2 fl.oz.	60 mL
1/2 cup	4 fl.oz.	120 mL
1 cup	8 fl.oz.	240 mL
1 1/2 cup	12 fl.oz.	355 mL
2 cups or 1 pint	16 fl.oz.	475 mL
4 cups or 1 quart	32 fl.oz.	1 L
1 gallon	128 fl.oz.	4 L

Temperatures Equivalents	
FAHRENHEIT(F)	CELSIUS(C) APPROXIMATE)
225 °F	107 °C
250 °F	120 ° °C
275 °F	135 °C
300 °F	150 °C
325 °F	160 °C
350 °F	180 °C
375 °F	190 °C
400 °F	205 °C
425 °F	220 °C
450 °F	235 °C
475 °F	245 °C
500 °F	260 °C

Weight Equivalents	
US STANDARD	METRIC (APPROXIMATE)
1 ounce	28 g
2 ounces	57 g
5 ounces	142 g
10 ounces	284 g
15 ounces	425 g
16 ounces (1 pound)	455 g
1.5 pounds	680 g
2 pounds	907 g

Appendix 2 The Dirty Dozen and Clean Fifteen

The Environmental Working Group (EWG) is a nonprofit, nonpartisan organization dedicated to protecting human health and the environment Its mission is to empower people to live healthier lives in a healthier environment. This organization publishes an annual list of the twelve kinds of produce, in sequence, that have the highest amount of pesticide residue-the Dirty Dozen-as well as a list of the fifteen kinds ofproduce that have the least amount of pesticide residue-the Clean Fifteen.

THE DIRTY DOZEN

The 2016 Dirty Dozen includes the following produce. These are considered among the year's most important produce to buy organic:

Strawberries	Spinach
Apples	Tomatoes
Nectarines	Bell peppers
Peaches	Cherry tomatoes
Celery	Cucumbers
Grapes	Kale/collard greens
Cherries	Hot peppers

The Dirty Dozen list contains two additional items-kale/collard greens and hot peppers- because they tend to contain trace levels of highly hazardous pesticides.

THE CLEAN FIFTEEN

The least critical to buy organically are the Clean Fifteen list. The following are on the 2016 list:

Avocados	Papayas
Corn	Kiw
Pineapples	Eggplant
Cabbage	Honeydew
Sweet peas	Grapefruit
Onions	Cantaloupe
Asparagus	Cauliflower
Mangos	

Some of the sweet corn sold in the United States are made from genetically engineered (GE) seedstock. Buy organic varieties of these crops to avoid GE produce.

Appendix 3 Index

A

almond 27, 30, 44
apple 26
apple cider vinegar 26
avocado 26, 39, 46, 49, 51, 52, 53, 58
avocado oil 39, 46, 49, 51, 52, 58

B

bacon 14, 15, 25, 26, 27, 38, 44, 51
baking soda 27, 29, 31
balsamic vinegar 45, 57
basil 23, 32, 38, 39, 47
bell pepper 25, 38, 55
broccoli 14, 16, 20
buns 44
butter 23, 24, 29, 30, 31, 33, 39, 40, 47

C

cauliflower 14, 32, 45, 51, 55, 59
cayenne 14, 18, 29, 32, 56, 59
cayenne pepper 23, 29, 32, 56, 59
Cheddar cheese 56
cheese 14, 19, 24, 25, 27, 29, 31, 32, 33, 34, 36
cinnamon 24, 29
coconut 26, 29, 31, 32, 40, 45, 49, 51, 52, 59
coriander 25, 57

cream 14, 16, 21, 24, 29, 30, 32, 33, 37, 40, 41, 46, 47, 55
cumin 59

D

Dijon mustard 25, 27, 47
dried rosemary 23

E

egg 25, 27, 30, 40, 49
Erythritol 30

F

flour 27, 31, 40, 49
fresh cilantro 34, 40, 46
fresh parsley 34, 46, 57
fruit 45

G

garlic 14, 15, 25, 31, 33, 36, 37, 39, 40, 44, 45, 46
garlic powder 14, 18, 45, 47, 58, 60

H

honey 58

J

juice 34, 43, 46, 50, 53, 56

K

kale 23, 56
kosher salt 30, 33, 41, 45, 47, 57, 60

L

lemon 43, 46, 50, 52, 53, 56
lemon juice 43, 46, 56
lime 34, 49, 53, 65
lime juice 34, 53

M

milk 26, 30, 32, 37, 51
Mozzarella 38
muffin 23, 27
mustard 25, 27, 43, 44, 47, 55, 58

N

nutmeg 60
nuts 56, 58, 59

O

oil 36, 37, 38, 39, 40, 43, 44, 45, 46, 49, 50
olive oil 36, 37, 40, 43, 44, 45, 50, 53, 55, 56
onion 25, 31, 37, 43, 47, 51, 52, 55

P

paprika 31, 36, 39, 44, 47, 58
Parmesan cheese 38, 60

parsley

parsley 34, 45, 46, 50, 57

R

red pepper flakes 25, 50, 55, 57
rice 59

S

salt 23, 25, 30, 31, 32, 33, 34, 37, 38, 39
sauce 36, 38, 40, 41, 45, 47, 49, 50, 51, 53, 57
sugar 45, 46, 49, 51, 53, 57

T

thyme 39, 52, 53
tomato 23, 24, 36, 38, 55
turmeric 37

V

vanilla 26, 29, 30, 32, 33
vegetable 39
vinegar 26, 40, 45, 52, 57

W

walnut 30

Y

yogurt 24, 29, 34

From Garden to Table | 65

Christina J. Williamson

Manufactured by Amazon.ca
Bolton, ON

40027171R00042